## PRAISE FOR VENUS ~~I~~

"At the end of the twentieth century~~...~~ your daughter may seem extremely tough—until you read Bartle and Lieberman. *Venus in Blue Jeans* is a welcome and useful guide for caring parenting in the post-virginal age."

—Joan Jacobs Brumberg, author of
*The Body Project: An Intimate History
of American Girls*

"Effective communication about these critically important topics is an art, not a science, and the practical wisdom contained in this book will help mothers—and fathers—meet the challenge."

—*Booklist*

"Mothers today know how important it is to speak openly to their daughters about sex. But what messages should they give? How do they begin a candid conversation? . . . Nathalie Bartle, with Susan Lieberman, throws valuable light on these questions. All parents will welcome *Venus in Blue Jeans,* for this book shows how we can impart information to our daughters and teach them about care and control in sexual matters, while we encourage them to have confidence in their own sexuality."

—Terri Apter, author of
*Altered Loves: Mothers and
Daughters During Adolescence*

"*Venus in Blue Jeans* fills a gap in the literature on adolescence: how mothers and daughters can talk about their thoughts and feelings about sexual development. From comprehensive interviews of mothers and daughters, Nathalie Bartle distills much wisdom for how parents can help girls move from childhood, through adolescence, to maturity."

—Julius Richmond, M.D., former U.S. surgeon general

"The voices of both generations of women are honest and forthright, and nullify many myths about the mother-daughter relationship. . . . Bartle writes from experience and her never-condescending voice reports and comments on her findings with authority. Her advice on opening and using lines of dyadic communication to shape the sexual choices of young women is frank, aware of differences in lifestyle, and caring."

—*Publishers Weekly*

## QUANTITY SALES

**Most Dell books are available at special quantity discounts** when purchased in bulk by corporations, organizations, or groups. Special imprints, messages, and excerpts can be produced to meet your needs. For more information, write to: Dell Publishing, 1540 Broadway, New York, NY 10036. Attention: Director, Special Markets.

## INDIVIDUAL SALES

**Are there any Dell books you want but cannot find in your local stores?** If so, you can order them directly from us. You can get any Dell book currently in print. For a complete up-to-date listing of our books and information on how to order, write to: Dell Readers Service, Box DR, 1540 Broadway, New York, NY 10036.

# Venus in Blue Jeans

## WHY MOTHERS AND DAUGHTERS
## NEED TO TALK ABOUT SEX

❈

## Nathalie Bartle, Ed.D.

*with Susan Lieberman, Ph.D.*

A Dell Trade Paperback

A DELL TRADE PAPERBACK

Published by
Dell Publishing
a division of
Random House, Inc.
1540 Broadway
New York, New York 10036

ISBN: 0-440-50880-0

Reprinted by arrangement with Houghton Mifflin Company

Printed in the United States of America

Published simultaneously in Canada

June 1999

10  9  8  7  6  5  4  3  2  1

*In memory of my mother,*
*Lurline Reaves Akin,*
*and for my daughter,*
*Katherine*

# Acknowledgments

I wish I could thank by name every mother and daughter who agreed to share something of their own relationships and experiences to make this book possible. For reasons of confidentiality, I cannot. Nevertheless, I will forever be grateful to all of these women for opening their minds and their hearts to me with the hope that their stories might help others. I also gratefully acknowledge the assistance I received from administrators, faculty, and staff at the two schools where my initial research was based.

I was most fortunate to have the wise and thoughtful guidance of faculty at Harvard's Graduate School of Education and School of Medicine as I worked on my dissertation, which provided the core research for this book. My special thanks to Julius B. Richmond, M.D., who untiringly and unselfishly assisted me with many aspects of my learning at Harvard and who continued to encourage and provide professional and personal support throughout the writing of this book. Having the opportunity to be mentored by Julie Richmond has been a great blessing in my life.

I am deeply appreciative of Professor Robert A. LeVine, who served as my adviser throughout my graduate program. Bob's sensible advice, his understanding of human development in all its fullness, and his belief in the importance of this book continued to be a source of inspiration. I also gratefully acknowledge the creative ideas, encouragement, and support I have received from Professor Carol Gilligan. This book first took shape in Carol's adolescent psychology course, and over a period of several years she has continued to support this work.

Professor Sara Lawrence Lightfoot, an inspiring teacher and researcher, provided her wisdom and guidance, and I am grateful to her.

Barrie Van Dyck, my agent, was a driving force behind my work. A real inspiration, she never faltered in her efforts to bring about the publication of this book. My thanks to Barrie for her understanding, encouragement, and friendship.

I wish especially to acknowledge Susan Lieberman's contributions to this work. She brought a fresh and creative pen to my research and writing as well as sage ideas to the content of the book. I am also indebted to Betsy Torg, who did an unbelievable job as my research assistant over the past eighteen months. Betsy was always willing to go the extra mile in tracking down information even as she carried out her responsibilities as a full-time student in the field of public health.

My colleagues and friends at Allegheny University of the Health Sciences School of Public Health, the Maternity Care Coalition, and the Office of Maternal and Child Health, all in Philadelphia, have been extremely helpful and encouraging. They unselfishly shared their time and expertise as I expanded my research and completed my writing. To them I express my appreciation.

I am thankful for the professional and personal support I received from my dear friends Cathy Gronewold and Edith Phelps. They were never too tired or too busy to listen, to offer ideas, and, finally, to read the full manuscript. To other colleagues and friends who held focus groups, who read the manuscript and provided supportive comments and encouragement I also say thank you: Paula Braverman, Hester Brooks, Robert Coles, Nancy Elfant, JoAnne Fischer, JoAnn Howard, Cherie Melino, Gail Murphy, Bob and Jan Randolph, Ann Smith, Chris Smith, Harold Straughn, Jim Taylor, and Marian Taylor.

Wendy Holt, my editor, was indefatigable in her support. Throughout the writing of this book she contributed her outstanding editing skills, her passion, her sensitivity, and her wisdom to help make it the best book possible. My deepest thanks to Wendy. It has been a delight to work with her and with my manuscript editor, Peg Anderson, as well as with other members of the Houghton Mifflin team.

And a heartfelt thanks to my family. The Akins — my loving, supportive parents (George and Lurline), my brother and sister (Bud and Kathy), and their families — and the Bartles, especially Louisa, Quartie, and Peter, have been behind me all the way on this project.

To my children and their spouses, Katherine and Bob and Jon and Christine, my two grandsons, Rex and James, and the voice of Jay, who kept saying "Go for it, Mom," I thank you for listening to me, laughing with me, and always loving me as you shared in the ups and downs of my writing. Katherine is at the heart of this book, and I am deeply grateful (and indebted) for her willingness to become a true partner on a project that we thought could help other mothers and daughters.

Finally, I want to acknowledge from the bottom of my heart the untiring and enthusiastic support I received from my husband from beginning to end. His wisdom, his questions, his humor, and his reading of draft after draft all contributed immeasurably to the final product. Harvey's constant encouragement and love have enabled me to write this book, and I am deeply thankful.

# Contents

........................................

## Afterword ❖ Beyond the Family

Involving the Community

## Appendix ❖ Organizations

# Venus in Blue Jeans

# ONE

# It's about Time

## NEW TIMES, NEW TALK

........❧........

W hen my children were old enough to entrust with a house key, they sometimes arrived home from school before I returned from work. At least one day a week, though, I would try to be there when they rushed through the front door, hoping they'd share some end-of-the-day news. Jon, then a freshman in high school, would often return late from after-school sports and, until he unwound, was generally oblivious to my presence. Jay, the youngest, was eleven and liked to talk at bedtime. After school he blew in, searched for food, and usually blew right back out to kick around a soccer ball with his friends. The child most likely to sit and talk with me was my twelve-year-old daughter, Katherine. If I caught Katherine at the right moment, she would talk easily about school, friends, and her feelings and ask the kind of wide-ranging questions that only a twelve-year-old would dream of.

On the days when Katherine attended a voluntary after-school sex education class for eighth-grade students at her junior high school, I made a point of getting home early just in case the class led us, as it often did, into an easy talking time. On one of those afternoons, I was in the kitchen slicing tomatoes for a dinner salad when I heard the front door slam. Without a word, my daughter tossed her backpack onto the couch, came into the kitchen, and headed for the refrigerator. After grabbing an apple, she plopped down on a chair at the kitchen table and launched into her description of sex education: "That class today was so gross! I can't believe they were talking to us about masturbation. That is *so* disgusting." My eyes stayed carefully focused on the tomato as my thoughts raced. How best to respond? I certainly didn't agree with Katherine, but how could I present a different, that is, a positive, perspective on masturbation? I remember being surprised at how uncomfortable I suddenly felt.

"Well," I began hesitantly, "masturbation doesn't have to be thought of as something so disgusting." Katherine looked stunned. "Come on," she said, "it's disgusting — people who sit around and play with themselves?" Thankful for the lettuce I was tearing into bits so I didn't have to look at her, I said, in what I hoped was a natural and relaxed tone, "Actually, it *can* be very nice; of course, masturbation is a pretty private thing, and . . . it's not something you do all the time."

I could feel her gaze weighing on me, could imagine her accusing look as she followed with the question, "Do *you* masturbate?" That lettuce pile was growing higher and higher. Part of me was glad my daughter felt comfortable enough to discuss masturbation with me, but another part was secretly wondering why I hadn't had the foresight to stay late at work that night. "Yes," I said quietly, "sometimes."

That was it for Katherine. She jumped up from her chair, grabbed her backpack from the couch, and headed down the hallway to her bedroom without looking back, shouting, "Gross. I can't believe my mother plays with herself." The bedroom door slammed shut.

What had I just done? Would Katherine never again touch herself? Would she lock her bedroom door and masturbate for hours at a time? Or would she now feel secret relief that touching herself was not, in fact, so outrageous? What was she going to think of me, her mother, after my confession? I wondered, How does a twelve-year-old relate to a mom she has just tagged as "someone who plays with herself"?

Should I have explained that she had unconsciously touched herself as a little girl or that masturbation was often the right first step for adolescents in exploring their sexuality? Should I have gone down the hall and knocked on her door or waited to see if this was the last conversation about sex we would have? The questions were overwhelming; what I did was take the easy way out. I moved on to slicing the green pepper, determined to make the most bountiful salad ever.

I had looked forward to these chats with Katherine, and I had certainly thought I'd be prepared to answer her questions. At the time I was an assistant professor in the pediatrics department at the University of Texas at Galveston Medical School, and I had spent many hours evaluating and counseling adolescents in our clinic. I was one of the faculty members who taught sexuality classes to medical students and had even helped to develop the sex education curriculum that Katherine's class was following. For many years I had been a counselor in public schools and private schools, and I had engaged teenage girls in conversations about a host of issues, including sexuality. I couldn't recall any of my students asking me directly about masturbation, but if they had, I was sure I would not have been fazed by the question. But now that my own daughter was moving into adolescence, where was that professional comfort level I had relied on so often? My older son's adolescence had not caused such uneasiness. What irony, I thought. I, the self-assured professional, was at a loss for what to say or do next. Suddenly my every word seemed to carry so much more meaning.

It was true that I had never felt comfortable discussing sex with my own mother, but I very much wanted Katherine to feel at ease talking with me about sexual topics. I had begun discussing anatomy with her as early as preschool. Yet now, suddenly, I was worried about divulging too much. I didn't want her to dismiss her mother as an oddball who masturbated every chance she got, but I also didn't want her to view her body and her sexuality as, to use her word, "gross." In the most personal way, I suddenly identified with all those parents I had talked with who were struggling to find ways to discuss sex that were effective for their children yet not fraught with anxiety for them.

The discomfort I experienced that day seemed to usher in a new period in which it became more and more difficult for me to talk with Katherine. As she was moving into her teens, I was moving into my forties. I felt a collision of emotions, which propelled me to revisit issues of my own adolescence, especially my relationship with my mother. She and I had skirted any discussions about sex in those years. In fact, the word "sex" hardly ever came up. She had great difficulty speaking this supposedly sinister word, and when she did, it sounded as though she were saying "sick." It was unimaginable that she would use the word "masturbation," let alone discuss it while slicing tomatoes.

In the 1950s in my conservative Christian community in north Texas, there were no confusing messages about sexual activity for girls because everyone simply delivered the same dictum: sex before marriage was wrong; it was a sin. If a girl felt "unnatural urges," she was supposed to sublimate them by playing sports or marching in the school band. Of course, no one discussed these urges, and watching Katherine grow up, I recalled my own feelings of adolescent confusion and loneliness. I had many friends, but none of us was able to articulate or even recognize the often painful challenges of adolescence. We were all too busy striving to be perfect and all too aware of our own shortcomings. Even later, at seventeen, when I was immensely attracted to a twenty-two-year-old boy I was dating, I broke up with him, too frightened to find out where my desire might take me, afraid of feelings I had been told were sinful. If I had turned to my mother for advice about sex and sexuality, I am sure I would have been disappointed. What my mother discussed with me — what was safe — was, among other things, how to make a good salad.

## A Legacy of Silence

Many years after my children were grown, I had a chance to discuss my memories with other women who shared this legacy of silence. In my first weeks as a graduate student in developmental psychology at Harvard, I became friends with three other women in Carol Gilligan's adolescent psychology class. All of us were middle-aged mothers of daughters, and we shared an interest in some of the recent research on the development of adolescent girls. One day at lunch the four of us were talking about an assignment that included stories by teenage girls on growing up. We discovered we all had the same urge to speak from a mother's perspective to the issues the girls were raising. What, we wondered, would the mothers of these girls think about what their daughters were saying? Would they disapprove, as the girls believed, or were the daughters projecting their own fears onto their moms? Did their mothers think they were doing a better or worse job of communicating their feelings and thoughts about sexual topics than their daughters perceived? And if the daughters opened the door to communication, would these moms want to reveal their own recollections of adolescence?

There at lunch was born the idea of organizing discussions with mothers of teenage girls. During the 1988–89 academic year, we conducted two focus groups (approximately eight women in each group), followed by individual interviews with forty women — single, married, and divorced — from diverse social, ethnic, and cultural backgrounds who had at least one adolescent daughter. We assembled the groups largely through our professional and personal acquaintance. For instance, the ten women I interviewed included African-American and white women from low-income and working-class neighborhoods. Another colleague interviewed middle- and upper-middle-class white mothers in two-parent families, while another interviewed white single-parent mothers. My Hispanic colleague interviewed Hispanic and white women from working- and middle-class neighborhoods.

Our purpose was to inquire generally about the relationship between mothers and their teenage daughters. We hoped to hear moms reflect on what it was like to raise an adolescent girl, what obstacles they encountered, what successes they had, and where they found support. We were interested in learning what mothers believed aided or disrupted communication with their daughters, what issues were important, and how they went about addressing those issues during the turbulent teenage years.

If our interests were general, the mothers' were more focused. They kept directing the discussion back to the specific subject of mother-daughter communication about sex and sexuality. They talked about the sudden changes that had occurred when their daughters began puberty and how their daughters' budding sexuality introduced conflicts to their relationships. They were concerned about the peer pressure on the girls to become sexually active and angry about the messages girls were receiving from friends and the media about how mature, hip, and even popular they would be if they had sex. They grappled with whether they should discuss birth control and, if so, what they should say.

Mothers were frightened that their teens would be exploited sexually by young men who falsely claimed care and commitment; they spoke, too, of feeling loss and even hurt as in midadolescence their daughters seemed to withdraw from them and close ranks with their peers. As their daughters made the transition from girlhood to womanhood, these moms felt that they too were in a transition period from the intense years of child rearing to a time of greater independence. Many women spoke about how a daughter's adolescence had stimulated their own growth and change, sometimes forcing a rethinking of values and expectations, in some cases leading them to become more aggressive in their own education or career endeavors. All of us, participants in the discussion sessions and leaders alike, valued the opportunity the talks afforded for reflection and reaffirmation. But in listening to the voices of moms, we four realized that in a somewhat ironic fashion we had come full circle in our thinking; we now found ourselves wondering what the daughters of these women would think if they had an ear to the wall.

We also began to notice an interesting pattern in the conversations with mothers. Often a woman would begin by telling the group a story about discussing sex with her daughter, but that story would soon segue into another vignette about a conversation or incident involving her own mother. Remembering the pull I had felt to look back, spurred by Katherine's adolescence, I was intrigued by this common impulse to turn to our relationships with our own mothers as a touchstone. The stories frequently began with these kinds of refrains: "My mother never discussed sex," "My mother could not deal with sexual issues," "My mother made sex such a dirty thing," "Sex was not discussed," "Nobody told me anything, "Menstruation was 'the curse' in my family," "My mother never had her period; she was always 'unwell.'"

Long after the legacy of silence is supplanted with experience and information, many grown women I spoke with missed their mothers' long-sought affirmation that their adolescent sexual selves, their seeking and inquiring selves, were legitimate and even desirable. In listening to the words women chose to recount their experiences and to the longing in their voices when they described how their mothers, like mine, had been silent, I was struck that even as grownups with children of our own, we still felt we had been cheated out of something important. Why did so many mature, seemingly confident women express this persistent sense of loss? This is the baggage and the history that moms today bring to their conversations with their daughters about sex. Thankfully, many of them are striving to break the legacy of silence with their own girls.

Because sex is so much with us, so much on the minds of adolescents and so much a part of a healthy adult life, not mentioning it is like ignoring an elephant in the kitchen. And who would ever argue that it *isn't* necessary to mention the elephant because everyone sees he's there or because we have no idea how to make him go away? By the same token, we need to talk about sex. We mention the vagaries of love frequently, yet love is more mysterious than sex. If we can reduce the feelings of incredible ignorance around sex that so many of us experienced growing up, just think how much more psychic space we'll create for our girls' thoughtful introspection. Rather than wondering about how they'll get the appropriate information, they can invest their energies in more engaging, value-driven questions.

Before declaring that it is impossible to address sexual intimacy with daughters, we might ask ourselves why. If our mothers never talked, do we look back on their silence with good feelings? If we are unsure about our feelings, might it be that expressing our confusion would help our daughters understand some of their own confusions? Could talking be a growing experience for both us and our girls?

I have come to understand that when moms and daughters talk

about sex, they are talking about far more than where babies come from or how to conduct themselves with boys. Our communication about sex deeply affects — and reflects — how we feel about the passage from girlhood to womanhood. And the way we feel about this passage, in turn, plays into how we communicate with our daughters. A mother's words may convey her ambivalence about losing her little girl while still wanting to welcome and accept the young woman she is becoming.

Communication about sexual topics may also initiate a shift in the power balance between mothers and daughters. Suddenly girls are on a more equal footing, where their thoughts and feelings are just as important and worthy of being heard as those of the mother.

Because conversation about sex incorporates all of the hopes, fears, joys, and uncertainties that mothers feel as their daughters begin their journey into womanhood and young adult relationships, it's understandable that it may make moms feel uncomfortable and that we may even wish to avoid discussing sex.

## Learning from Mother-Daughter Pairs

By the end of the academic year, the women I was working with and I had learned an enormous amount about mother-daughter communication and concerns, but many questions remained unanswered. I was more interested than ever in hearing mothers and daughters from the same families speak about particular issues. And, given the mothers' earlier emphasis on communication about sex, it was a natural next step to choose for further research the topic of mother-daughter communication about sex. I decided to interview a diverse group of mother-daughter pairs so that I would get to hear both speak to the same questions. With the help of two schools, one an inner-city public high school and the other a private suburban precollegiate school, I was able to conduct comprehensive interviews with twenty-three mother-daughter pairs from different social environments and economic levels and of different races and ethnicities.

Many times during my interviews I found myself wishing these conversations had occurred years earlier, before my own daughter approached adolescence. Had I been able to consult with these moms and girls when Katherine and I were hitting bumps on the rocky road of her adolescence, I am confident it would have been an easier, happier time for both of us. Other women I talked to had similar responses. When the nature of these interviews came up in conversation, friends, colleagues, or mothers I was meeting for the first time always asked what I had learned: what was working in communication and what wasn't, what could they draw on to strengthen their own relationships with their girls?

There is no quick and simple recipe to ensure that sharing our feelings about sex will go smoothly. Yet one theme that first appeared in those early discussion groups reappeared in later conversations: mothers were determined to "do it differently," to "do it better" than their own moms had. Moms, though confused as to how best to go about it, wanted to help their daughters learn about sexuality and all the joys and potential dangers wrapped up in it.

Alma Parks, one of the mothers interviewed, spoke with deep regret about her own mother's silence. When she was growing up, Alma wished her mother had "just talk[ed] with me and [told] me about womanly things. It wasn't discussed. It was just like these things were so bad, and I thought to myself maybe if I had been taught some things and my mother related to me as a mother . . . I don't think I would have made some wrong choices early in my life."

There never was much love in Alma's marriage, which began when she was in high school, but with no job skills and a young child, she believed her only choice was to stay. When she finally left the marriage and began to pursue a college degree, she had the chance to seek out life's other pleasures. "But if someone had been teaching and talking to me, I would have been able to fulfill these things years ago," she said. As a result, Alma was insistent on guarding her daughters from similar hardships. "We talk . . . and I talk seriously. I don't play, and I don't beat around the bush," she said. "I use myself as an example."

Another mother, Phyllis Rosenbloom, recalled with bemusement her most important sex education conversation with her mother. "I was twenty when I got married. My mother had never discussed sex with me, but the night before my wedding, she sort of tiptoed into my room and told me she just wanted me to know one thing: 'Sex gets better.' It wasn't much of an education but at least she was accurate." Phyllis, however, had been answering her own daughters' questions about sex since her oldest daughter turned five. She both initiated conversations and responded to her girls' questions, although at times she worried, like many a mother, that she was "not doing a very good job at this."

Not all of the mothers, of course, had had unsatisfactory or unfulfilling experiences learning about their sexuality. One psychotherapist, now with two daughters of her own, remembered getting her first period and calling her mother at work to announce the event. "My parents closed the store and came home together to take me out to dinner to celebrate the joy of becoming a woman. We celebrated in the same way with each of our daughters." Usually, however, when I mentioned that I was interested in how mothers communicate with daughters about sex, positive stories were much less frequent than the two words I was to hear over and over: "What communication?"

In all of the discussions with mothers who recalled their own sex education, I never encountered one who said, "My mother didn't speak with me about it. That worked well, and that's the tack I'm going to take with my daughter." Rather, they were all making marked efforts to do right by their daughters, and most believed they were doing a much better job than their own moms when it came to open and direct communication. Why was it, then, that some of the girls echoed their mothers' own words: "What communication?"

## Everyone Tells and No One Tells

America has a cultural split personality when it comes to discussing sex. On the one hand, we view sex as deeply private and consider it a subject of great intimacy. A teacher in a small town in New Mexico, for instance, once told me that her district forbade even using the word "sex" in sex education classes. On the other hand, we talk about sex everywhere all the time — in newspapers, magazines, movies, on television and in cyberspace, on the faces of billboards and on the backsides of cabs. What can it mean to a teenager when a word can't be spoken in sex education class but is seen and heard everywhere else? Teenagers must see in this odd circumspection more hypocrisy than morality. Surely it models the acceptability of teaching one thing and doing another.

Such inconsistencies arose in my own work from time to time. At the University of Texas, where I was part of a teaching team on human sexuality for freshman medical students, students and faculty clashed continuously over whether this class was an essential element of the curriculum or an unnecessary nuisance. On the day when we were supposed to discuss homosexuality, some students refused to participate. For other students the course material triggered difficult personal questions. A young woman who had been married for several years asked to meet with me after class one day. It turned out she didn't want to discuss test scores but instead wanted to know exactly what an orgasm was and how she would know if she had had one. Although this incident occurred several years ago, I feel that intelligent young women today still do not always possess the necessary knowledge to deal effectively and wisely with the pressures, perversions, or pleasures of sexuality they may be confronted with, and silence does little to prepare them.

Oddly enough, eighth-graders in our local school in Galveston seemed less inhibited than my medical students when it came to talking about sex. When my youngest son, Jay, was in eighth grade, he came home one day announcing he had won his sex education class contest. When I asked him what the contest was for, he proudly reported, "I came up with the longest list of slang terms for the word 'penis.'" I couldn't decide if Jay's facility meant I was a success or a failure as a parent. Despite Jay's enthusiasm for the class, some parents had requested that their children be excused from it.

Such stories, I think, hint at an underlying confusion in our society about how to handle sex education. Teens believe they know a great deal about sex, and we believe that they do, too. Yet their knowledge is usually selective and incomplete, often shaped by the media and by peers' accounts. The teen pregnancy rate in the United States is twice as high as in England, Wales, and Canada; three times as high as in Sweden and Norway; and more than seven times as high as in the Netherlands. When asked about sexually transmitted diseases (STDs), many teens mention only AIDS — acquired immunodeficiency syndrome. Most of the girls I interviewed did not think abortion was legal.[1]

We make the mistake of thinking that saying words that convey our feelings will lead to actions. If we tell our children about intercourse and contraception, we fear they will have sex. If we tell them about masturbation, we fret that they may develop self-destructive behaviors. If we tell them about orgasm, we worry they won't be able to resist temptation. All too often we *don't* talk, believing that silence or directives without dialogue are protective strategies. But we are not protecting our children from sex; we are protecting them from context. For teens, this approach falls dangerously short. In this culture teenagers already know a great deal about intercourse and condoms, masturbation, oral and anal sex.[2] What they don't know and need to learn is how to process the information, how to apply what they do know to various situations, and how to interpret information from different sources that may seem at cross-purposes. They require our help in understanding sex in the broader context of relationships and sexuality in the context of normal adolescent development.

That teens aren't receiving this kind of critical guidance was driven home for me by my involvement with the Maternity Care Coalition (MCC) of Philadelphia. A dynamic organization known throughout the region for its programs that aid mothers and children, MCC each year sponsors a conference on an issue of special concern to professionals in the field of maternal and child health as well as to parents, adolescents, politicians, religious leaders, and teachers. The topic for 1996 was "Pregnant Pause: Time to Talk about Teens, Sex and the Next Generation." To prepare for the conference, the planning committee held discussion groups with urban, suburban, and rural teens from southeastern Pennsylvania. The goal was to explore what a diverse group of adolescent boys and girls were thinking about some key sexual topics and to determine if teens from different communities shared common concerns.

Approximately two hundred students from widely different socio-economic backgrounds participated. Some were pregnant or were already parents. We posed to them a number of questions, including these: What does it feel like to be a teenager today? Whom do you talk to about sex? What topics do you discuss with your mother? With your father? Whom else do you talk with about sex? What influences your thoughts and decisions about whether to become sexually active?[3]

In listening to them describe how they learned about sexuality, we found that they believed they had learned very little from their parents. For example, when we asked how teens learn about sex today, they told us, "Not from parents or adults. . . . It's a myth that parents tell kids about sex." Parents, both boys and girls reported, were afraid of talking about sex and uncomfortable raising issues related to sexual behavior. What's more, these teens shared their parents' discomfort in addressing sexual issues. Discussion about sex, they said, was most likely to occur when their parents used "sound bites" from television shows to make a point or start a conversation. Some of the boys and girls reported talking with their moms about sex, but they said it "felt awkward." They preferred short conversations that provided information and avoided questions. Dads, we heard, were not the ones to consult. This sentiment was equally true for boys and girls. Fathers, most girls reported, ignored daughters' emerging sexuality or just said, "Don't do it — don't get pregnant."

These comments, though they underscore the challenges for both parents and teens, must be taken in perspective. Teens are reluctant to praise parents in public; this is definitely uncool behavior. And mid-adolescence tends to be the low point in parent-teen communication.

Despite these youthful protestations about the irrelevance of parents, most research supports our parental instincts: we are far from irrelevant in our teenagers' lives. In a recent survey of some 90,000 adolescents, researchers examined what really works to discourage teens from engaging in high-risk behaviors such as smoking marijuana or cigarettes, drinking, or having sex. Their results indicated, overwhelmingly, that a close-knit family was the key factor.[4] Other studies reveal that parents' *talking* about sex with their children can serve as a deterrent to teens' having sex, or, if they should become sexually active, these teens are more likely to use contraception.

Nancy Chodorow's work further demonstrates that the mother-daughter relationship is one of the most primary of all attachments. As I discovered, no book, computer, or videocassette, no class or peer group is as strong an influence on a young daughter's understanding of and attitude toward sex as her mother.[5] Added to all of this is the compelling evidence of mature women who still speak with regret about the lack of communication with their mothers about sex when they were growing up. Nor should fathers be left out of the picture; rather, they make up a largely untapped resource for helping us do a better job with sex education. Many fathers have yet to appreciate the important role they can play in maintaining adolescent girls' self-esteem during this stormy period.

## What Do We Say? When Do We Say It?

While most mothers are committed to ending the silence enveloping discussion of female sexuality, many find it more difficult than they anticipated to address sexual matters with their daughters. Part of the difficulty comes from changing community standards. Without widespread societal agreement, many mothers are unsure just what they should communicate. Some of us, reluctant to recall our own teenage behaviors, may rely instead on those very messages we found contradictory in our youth. Mothers who were sexually active as teens may want their daughters to remain abstinent but find that discussing sexuality calls to mind stories they prefer to keep hidden from their children — and even from themselves. Women who harbor secrets they consider shameful may feel especially vulnerable in talking with teenagers who have no idea what subjects trigger painful memories. Mothers who were sexually assaulted, especially as girls, may also be drawn to silence.

Secrets from the past came up in more than a few of my conversations with mothers. One talked about the conflicts she and her daughter were experiencing and confided that, unknown to her daughter, she'd become sexually active as a teen and regretted it. While she thought she was being open and direct with her daughter, the daughter described her as "unreasonably afraid that every contact with boys will lead to sex" and felt that it was "too dangerous" to ask her mom any questions.

Many parents are caught between their wishes and hopes for their daughters and the realities of adolescence in our culture. Most mothers with whom I spoke hoped their teenage daughters would delay sexual intimacy until after high school; a few advocated waiting until marriage. They worried about pregnancy and disease, emotional disequilibrium and loss of focus. Yet the reality is that 22 percent of fifteen-year-old girls have engaged in sexual intercourse, and some 65 percent of eighteen-year-olds have had sex.[6] It is exceedingly difficult for most parents to imagine that their teenage daughters are ready for sex physically or emotionally, yet the evidence suggests that girls are engaging in sexual intercourse nevertheless.

In my interviews, no mother was willing to admit that her daughter might be sexually active, even when the daughter suspected that her mother knew she was. While moms may believe they are far more forthright than their own mothers in saying, "When you're ready for sex, come talk with me and we will do something," their daughters more often report, "She won't discuss sex with me." Some mothers plan to have specific conversations with their daughters, but sometimes they delay these talks until it is too late. Four of every ten sexually active girls become pregnant before they reach the age of twenty — most of them — 80 percent — unintentionally. One in five of these girls will not use any contraception, while others use contraception irregularly.[7]

Effective communication about sex hinges on the temperament of each mother and each daughter and a daughter's age, interests, and physical and emotional development. Every discussion needs to be tailored to the girl's development and circumstances. For the majority of mothers and daughters I spoke with, however, the more comfortable the mother was in discussing sex and sexuality and listening to her daughter talk, the more at ease the daughter felt in broaching these subjects.

But there's that larger question: When the conversation is about sex, what should we be discussing? There is the hardware information — all the body parts related to sexuality and the mechanics of how those parts work, alone and with a partner. In the preschool and early school-age years, girls are curious about the differences between girls and boys and, eventually, about where babies come from. Soon it is time to explain menstruation, contraception, and disease prevention. Whispered words and raucous jokes provoke curiosity, and kids want to know what it all means. Not a few mothers have recalled, with a mixture of humor and dread, their struggles to respond to "What is fellatio?" "How do you have sex with an animal?" "How do women have sex together? "Do men really put their penises in women's mouths?" "Can you get AIDS from French kissing?"

Such questions tend to arrive when we're least expecting them, and, as I found with Katherine, we're not always prepared, despite our best intentions. If, as one mother described, the question comes zinging from the back of the car in rush-hour traffic, we may find ourselves gripping the wheel to avoid swerving from surprise. How we respond to these unexpected questions, however, is very important. It is one thing to say to a daughter "I have to think about the right way to answer that question," and quite another to say "That is not a question you should be asking" or "What made you ask that question?"

Different mothers use different strategies. A mother in St. Louis drives her daughter to a gynecologist to receive birth control; a mom in Houston shepherds her child to church to sign a chastity pledge. Not surprisingly, the outcomes of different responses vary, and the outcomes are not always consistent with parents' values. A loving couple in Boston that always delivered a clear and consistent message of abstinence, reinforced by their church, find themselves deeply pained to learn that their eighteen-year-old daughter is sexually active. Parents in San Diego with liberal sexual views are amazed when their twenty-two-year-old daughter advocates the virtues of virginity until she and her fiancé are married.

This book is not about which "right" is more right. It does not profess to offer a set of rules to ensure that every daughter will act just as we want her to. Rather, this book draws largely from the stories of a selected group of mothers and daughters, so it offers that particular window onto communication about sexuality. My hope is that we will be able to draw from what these teenagers and their mothers have to say and discover ideas about how we might best deal with these issues in our own families. It has always been my firm belief that the narratives we tell each other are the source of some of our richest insights. Perhaps the candid views of these moms and daughters — highlighting their knowledge, hopes, frustrations, and confusions — can be a catalyst for a nationwide conversation about sex and sexuality.

After interviewing mothers and daughters, I came away feeling that it is more important to be honest about our confusions than to pretend we are sure when we're not. Our girls read our ambivalence in neon and know from the undertones of our voices when our messages are not genuine. When we deceive our daughters, even if we believe we are distorting the truth "for their own good," we confuse them. Clear, open communication is the key to helping teenagers determine their own moral stance, but we have to embrace both "clear" and "open." A one-way lecture that is clear and closed or mixed messages about sexuality that are open but confusing don't succeed.

Whether mothers speak with words or with body language — which girls usually understand as well as declarative sentences — a mother's feelings become a reference point for a daughter in her growing-up years. We now understand that girls learn to define themselves not simply in individual terms but in the context of their relationships.[8] They judge themselves by their ability to care for those relationships, and they react strongly to detachment, indifference, or lack of concern from family and other loved ones. They strive to make their own voices heard and recognized, but they do not wish the cost to be abandoning either family or those they care about in relationships beyond the family. The message of this book is that we must remain connected and in a conversation that allows both daughters and mothers to be heard.

## All Our Daughters Are at Risk

Every teenage girl, no matter where she lives, is growing up in a risky time. A 1995 Carnegie Council report on adolescent development warned that across America, adolescents are confronting pressures to use alcohol, cigarettes, or other drugs and to have sex at earlier ages. The distressing report continued, "By age seventeen, about a quarter of all adolescents have engaged in behaviors that are harmful or dangerous to themselves and others: getting pregnant, using drugs, taking part in antisocial activity, and failing in school. Altogether, nearly half of American adolescents are at high or moderate risk of seriously damaging their life chances."

With a worried eye toward earlier sexual activity, the report stated, "Rates of sexual initiation are increasing among younger girls and boys. Many American teenagers are startlingly ignorant of the most elementary facts of the human body and human sexuality, despite their wholesale exposure to sex in the mass media, the availability of sexually related materials, and efforts to provide sexuality education in the schools."[9]

Given the urgency of the council's report and what we know from our own lives, it behooves us to reach out to girls so that they are able to make intelligent choices about and within their relationships, to feel proud of their bodies and their minds, and to become healthy, confident young women who appreciate their sexuality as one of the many satisfying components of womanhood.

Our daughters are wired for desire — and we probably wouldn't want it otherwise. Desire can be activated by a touch or a thought, a picture or a word. It is impossible to police all the stimuli that activate desire, and the more the sources of stimulation multiply, the harder control becomes. Rather than ignore desire or label it as something improper, we can acknowledge its normalcy and help our daughters understand how to manage desire rather than be shamed by or defiant with it.

"Sex" is a great, rich, complicated word. Metaphorically, it is a descriptive adjective that defines who we are; a noun that describes an endless array of people, places, and things; and a verb that conjures up activities that people all over the world find pleasurable. More than a word, it is a topic sentence for dissent and political posturing. It is a plot for complicated stories of interaction and intrigue, sometimes in our own families. It is a hypothesis for experimentation and curiosity. It is the grist of advertising copywriters, poets, and novelists. We desire sex, we deplore it, we regret it, or we do it, but whatever our stance, it remains on our minds. So it is natural that it will be on the minds of our daughters as they mature and begin to wonder how to relate to the opposite sex, or, in the case of those who already know by adolescence that they are lesbians, how to relate to other women romantically. We may avoid talking about sex, but there is no avoiding sexuality.

The chief executive officer of Planned Parenthood of Southeastern Pennsylvania wrote recently in a letter to the *Philadelphia Inquirer*, "Instead of providing responsible sex education for our youth, we offer them titillating advertising that uses sex to sell everything from toothpaste to clothes to cars. And then we blame them, the children we raise in ignorance, for not handling their sexuality and its consequences in a way that doesn't embarrass or shame or shock or sadden us."[10] This untenable situation can end with this generation if we as women will now speak with passion and honesty to our daughters, nieces, godchildren, and other special girls in our lives, if we will say, "I want you to know all that I can tell you about this wonderful but complicated subject of sex. Let's talk and puzzle this out together so I can help you grow into a woman who uses her good sense to arrive at good relationships that one day will lead to good sex." Then, I believe, when our adult daughters are asked, "How did you and your mother communicate about sex?" they will not respond wistfully or angrily,

"What communication?" They will say to their daughters, "My mother wasn't the perfect communicator, but she always believed it was important for us to talk about sex and sexuality. At times I didn't think it was a good idea, and I think she felt unsure and a little embarrassed. Now I understand why she persevered with me on this topic, and I want to do the same with you."

# TWO

# Parallel Worlds

## THE GIRLS OF JEFFERSON AND

## NOTTINGHAM HIGH SCHOOLS

I'd been warned that the massive front doors of Jefferson High School were bolted as soon as the 7:30 A.M. bell rang for the first class period. I cleared the metal detectors with just a few minutes to spare and picked up the pace of Jefferson students as they headed toward class. The students displayed every skin tone and every conceivable approach to fashion. Cornrows and curls, long red tresses and close-cropped crews, high-heeled sandals and purple Nikes swished by me. The kids were attractive, colorful, full of life — and loud. Then the bell rang. As if by magic, only the security guards, two administrators with walkie-talkies and I were left in the empty hall.*

My graduate-school colleagues and I were at Jefferson to provide part-time counseling services to students through a neighborhood health center grant. We gathered in the office of Jim Williams, the principal, who had been given the daunting job of merging two high schools with competing gangs to accommodate budget cuts. The two-year-old mega-school was located in a converted canning factory in a neighborhood marked by violence. Over the coming months we watched, often in disbelief, as Jim balanced the competing demands

---

*The schools, which are in an eastern city, and the mothers, daughters, and their stories are all real. However, I have changed names and other identifying information to protect the privacy of all those involved. The words of the mothers and daughters have not been changed except as necessary to disguise their identities.

of students, faculty, community, police, and parents with grace and guarded optimism. "We have more than our share of kids who need lots of help," he told us that first day. "But you will find most of the kids at Jefferson interested in learning and contributing to the school."

Nina Flynn, the director of Student Support Services, talked with us at greater length about the 1,300 students in grades nine through twelve: 80 percent of the student body qualified for the federally assisted lunch program; two hundred girls were already parents; fifty of their infants or toddlers were cared for in the school's daycare center. Teen moms whose children couldn't be accommodated there had to make outside arrangements for daycare if they wanted to return to school. Despite these tremendous obstacles, Nina was quick to point to the academic and other achievements of Jefferson students, many of whom came from "dysfunctional families." As I was to discover during my time as a counselor at the school, "dysfunctional" was a broad term that could mean anything from a father in jail and a mother on drugs to physical or emotional abuse or financial despair. Although the odds for future success were not in the students' favor, I was amazed at their resiliency and persistent determination to make the most of the opportunities they did have.

The school day at Jefferson ended at 1:30 P.M., when the building emptied and was again locked, but until then every minute was accounted for. Students had one thirty-minute break for lunch and only three minutes to move between classes before the halls were "swept" and stragglers dispatched to the "time-out room." Bathrooms were kept locked; keys had to be obtained from the counselors' offices. The coach of Jefferson's championship basketball team told us that when the student body was polled, 50 percent named gang violence as the most pressing problem in their lives. Killings and arrests were commonplace in the neighborhood. Although Jefferson had a fine interscholastic sports program in football, basketball, track, and baseball, only a small percentage of students was able to participate. Few intramural programs were available, and most of the programs in the fine arts and music had been eliminated.

With inadequate support staff, the counselors felt overworked and often frustrated, but it was clear they wanted their students to succeed. As one counselor explained, "If the kids we see have just one person in their lives who cares about them, they can make it." She talked with glowing pride about one young man who had become president of the student council and a valued member of the football team after the staff had worked intensively with him as a freshman. Yet she knew there was not enough time in any one week to focus on all the adolescents who needed support. When I announced my plan to interview mothers and daughters from Jefferson for a study of communication about sex, I understood it would mean more work for an already overburdened staff. Still, Jim Williams and the counselors were quick to offer support and encouragement, believing that sex education was an important issue for teens and parents.

### Nottingham Secondary School

In the thirty-five minutes it took to drive from the inner-city streets around Jefferson to the leafy green suburbs of Nottingham, the private school from which I was choosing mothers and daughters to talk with, I felt I was leaving one continent and arriving in another. I would pull in through Nottingham's gates in the late spring afternoon, when Jefferson's bleak fortress was locked cold and see well-dressed students everywhere. Nottingham had worked to diversify the student body, and about a fourth of the students were receiving some scholarship assistance, but the majority of students and faculty were white, conservatively dressed, and relatively affluent. Tuition at Nottingham was as much as some Jefferson parents earned in a year. Backed by an impressive thirteen-million-dollar endowment, the tuition bought a low student-faculty ratio, attractive grounds, and an attentive administration.

In the spring, girls and boys in grades seven through twelve chatted on the lawns between the school's several buildings after classes, or practiced lacrosse or soccer on the fields or shot baskets in the gym. Other students might be rehearsing a play in the theater, working on a science project in the lab, doing research in the airy library, or heading off for a community service project. On one afternoon visit the art director shepherded me through the studios to show off the students' artwork. It was not uncommon for Nottingham students to be at school until 5:30 or 6:00 P.M. every school day before going home to several hours of homework. The school day was structured, but students were free to travel in the halls to seek out a teacher.

With rare exceptions, all graduates went on to accredited four-year colleges and universities. Portraits of distinguished alumni, many of whose names were familiar because of their leadership roles at the state or national level, lined the corridor leading to the headmaster's office. Ben Smith, the headmaster, had begun his career at Nottingham as a young history teacher, and he conveyed a deep affection for both the students and the school. In just a few minutes of conversation he made it clear that he loved what he was doing. Nottingham seemed a vibrant, happy place, nurtured by strong relationships between faculty and students. I couldn't help but think that some of that happiness surely derived from the safety and serenity the school offered its students.

## Shared Visions

Looking at these two schools, one sees striking differences on the surface. But when I had the opportunity to talk intimately with mothers and daughters from Nottingham and Jefferson, what stood out, in fact, were the many similarities among the mother-daughter pairs. For all the disparities in their neighborhoods, school facilities, and family financial circumstances, mothers from both schools wanted the same things for their girls, and they shared many of the same fears. The Nottingham families may have lived in more lavish houses on safer streets, yet they were hardly free from worry about their daughters. Their fears were more abstract, perhaps, but every mother had concerns about her daughter's safety, sexual predators, and her girl's health and happiness. It was no easier to teach a daughter about sex in the suburbs than in the city. Nor was it any easier for an adolescent girl to confide in an affluent mother than in a working-class mom.

Education and broad experience may have helped some Nottingham mothers find the words to express their feelings and articulate their thoughts, yet these assets did not foster any more confidence that they were communicating effectively with their daughters about sex, nor did mothers' higher education ensure they would do a better job. Most of the Nottingham girls were more socially adept than the girls from Jefferson, but they did not always have greater or equal confidence, more curiosity, or more maturity to deal with sexual issues or the many other concerns of their adolescent lives. In fact, Jefferson girls were handling a whole host of responsibilities — such as taking care of siblings, holding jobs, and paying for life's basic necessities — that Nottingham girls couldn't imagine.

## Choosing Mother-Daughter Pairs

Sex is not a safe subject for schools. To allow a researcher, outside of the regular channels of school controls, to interact with students and parents on a study that asks explicit questions about sex, requires a school administrator with ample faith in his judgment as well as strong relationships with the students and parents. Still, both schools opened their doors willingly. It was the mothers and daughters who agreed to reveal their intimate thoughts and interactions, though, who showed the greatest courage.

The girls first completed a questionnaire at school that evaluated their communication with their mothers (or guardians) on a scale ranging from "open" to "problematic." One hundred and fifteen girls — sixty-five at Nottingham and fifty at Jefferson — completed questionnaires; their ages ranged from thirteen to seventeen, with the mean age being fourteen. The mothers were sent a parallel questionnaire to fill out; just under 40 percent of the girls' mothers returned completed questionnaires. With this information I could gauge the diversity of the mother-daughter pairs and decide whom to interview. When all the interviews were completed, the mothers and then the daughters from each of the schools were invited to participate in a final focus group.[1]

In some cases a girl was willing to participate but her mother was hesitant. One enthusiastic student from Jefferson desperately wanted her mom to be a part of the study, but each time we set an appointment, the mother called to cancel. Finally she told me she just couldn't find the time to participate; I suspect many mothers were uncomfortable risking scrutiny of their communication strategies.

In other cases the mother was enthusiastic and the daughter was reluctant. The girls, especially, were concerned about confidentiality. Many felt it was simply unsafe to speak honestly about sex to an adult, in most cases someone they did not know, who was going to be interviewing their mother. More than once, daughters would begin our interview by asking, "Now it's for sure that you are not going to tell my mother what I say, right?" It was a trust I worked hard to earn. Some of the girls, however, responded in the opposite way: they felt more comfortable talking to an adult they didn't know and were eager to talk nonstop. One girl observed that she felt more at ease talking about sexual issues in our interview than she could ever imagine feeling with her mother.

In the end, twenty-three mother-daughter pairs — twelve from Nottingham and eleven from Jefferson High School — signed on to be interviewed. At Jefferson five of these families were white, and six were African-American. The average age of the daughters was fifteen, and the mothers' average age was forty-one. The family annual incomes ranged from $15,000 to $50,000. Of the twelve pairs from Nottingham, seven were white, including one family in which the mother was Asian and the father Caucasian, and the other five were African-American. The average age of the daughters at Nottingham was fourteen, and the mothers' ages averaged to forty-three. The annual reported family income of the Nottingham families ranged from $40,000 to $300,000.

Each of the mothers and daughters met with me separately at the home, workplace, or school, and the interviews quickly took on the tenor of intimate conversations. The mothers especially were thoughtful, self-revealing, and quick to laugh. They spoke of their relationships with their own mothers, their teenage sexual experiences, their husbands and lovers, and particularly their daughters. Though I posed specific questions, often the interviewer/interviewee relationship evolved into one in which we were comrades in arms, strangers whose strangeness was set aside by our common bond as mothers. At the kitchen table or in an office conference room, we tackled collectively the mystery of our daughters' passage from girlhood to womanhood.

The girls were of all types. Some were articulate and confident; others were shy, still awkward with their bodies and sometimes with their thoughts, but possessing a certain fresh grace. Some were pretty by conventional standards; others had their own kind of beauty, which appeared when they smiled or their eyes lit up with a realization about themselves. Some girls chatted easily with no prodding at all, while others had to stretch to find their own voices, to give me answers they thought I wanted to hear.

These mothers and daughters presented many different approaches to talking about sex, from poor communication to direct and open discussion. What they had in common was their willingness to speak about this topic with someone else and their strong desire to talk with each other effectively about sexual issues.

## The Mothers and Daughters

The bond between mother and daughter is strong but elastic. I imagine it as made of gossamer woven with steel filaments, securing the rarest of relationships — complicated, changing, yet unbreakable. The girls were always in their mothers' sphere of influence, but they were much more than their mothers' creations. When a mother and her daughter responded to the same questions about their communications around sex, different pictures frequently emerged.

While there are tales here from a variety of mothers and daughters in focus groups, counseling sessions, and, sometimes, unexpected encounters, most of the stories in these pages come from the mother-daughter pairs at Jefferson and Nottingham, fifteen of which are highlighted. These fifteen were chosen to reflect different stages of adolescent development and to represent diverse views. Black and white, rich and poor, religious and nonreligious families thus illuminate a host of issues about discussing sex.

Here is a brief introduction to these fifteen.

### Mary Robbins and Vicki
### Evelyn Shepherd and Ingrid

Thirteen-year-old Vicki Robbins and Ingrid Shepherd, fourteen, were friends at Nottingham, and they shared that refreshing "the glass-is-half-full" approach to life. Both were the only children of involved professional parents who tried to talk often and easily with their curious daughters about sex and sexuality.

Vicki's mother, Mary Robbins, was a lawyer with a sophisticated but welcoming demeanor. She and Vicki lived in a condominium near Mary's office, but during the week Vicki boarded at Nottingham. Mary and Vicki's father had been divorced for nearly a decade. Still, Mel Robbins remained involved in Vicki's life, though he had recently moved to another city.

Ingrid's mom, Evelyn, was a straightforward, articulate woman who had taught school in many countries around the world for the military and had married late. She now ran a small part-time business from her home and thus was easily available for her daughter. The Shepherds were very committed to their "onliest child," and both parents gave Ingrid a great deal of attention. Dave Shepherd, Evelyn's dad and a business executive, was an active participant in his daughter's upbringing and liked to be a part of discussions that concerned Ingrid.

Physically, Vicki and Ingrid were opposites. Ingrid, though she was short, was developmentally precocious, and had gotten her first bra in third grade. Now, at the age of fourteen, she had begun to attract the attention of boys. Vicki was large for her age, slightly chubby, and just beginning to show signs of puberty. She was still more fireplug than shapely female and was not yet drawing boys' stares. Ingrid was by far the most curious and confident of the girls I talked with, and her mother seemed the most adept at presenting information in ways that were both matter-of-fact and easy for her daughter to understand.

### Cybil Mason and Bettina

Cybil Mason looked too young to be the mother of a thirteen-year-old. Easy to talk with, she was warm, outgoing, and thoughtful about how she wanted to raise Bettina. Bettina's dad and Cybil had divorced when Bettina was four, and although Dan Mason contributed both financially and emotionally to Bettina's upbringing, Cybil felt she had the primary responsibility in raising her daughter. Her experience as a teacher also gave her a detailed understanding of the stages of children's development, and she was trying to phase in information about sex as Bettina became ready for it. Still, Cybil worried that Bettina was too sheltered and wouldn't develop the street smarts to protect herself "in the real world." As a single mom, she had seen firsthand what the dating world was like for older women, and she was anxious about teenage dating.

In contrast to her mother, Bettina, a Nottingham student, appeared diffident and tentative. She brightened up most when she talked about her dream of skiing in the Olympics before settling down to a "serious career" but was hesitant to talk about her feelings in most other areas. I knew from her mother that Bettina was a good student, a talented writer, and an active participant in many extracurricular activities, but she was a reluctant self-promoter when we spoke.

### Rosemary Zimmerman and Erica

Like Bettina, fourteen-year-old Erica Zimmerman received good grades and had divorced parents. There the similarities stopped. Erica's soft features belied a down-home, outspoken manner. Four-letter words were a well-used part of her vocabulary, and her talk had a toughness that was hard to ignore. Her life had been more difficult than the lives of most of the girls I met with.

Erica's parents had divorced when she was ten, and she and her sister had lived with their mom. Her mother, however, had remarried a man who verbally and emotionally abused the girls, creating a volatile situation at home. One day Erica exploded with rage, and the family found itself in juvenile court. Ultimately the girls went to live with Erica's dad, whom she adored, but when he was arrested for stealing, the court placed the girls with their father's sister, Rosemary. Erica acknowledged that her aunt had taken them in when they had no other place to go but foster care, but theirs was not a warm or connected relationship.

Rosemary Zimmerman was a weary woman who cared for a sick mother, babysat for her grandchildren, and worried about how to provide for her nieces in a small apartment in one of the city's worst neighborhoods. She was trying to care responsibly for the girls but found them "disrespectful and troublesome." Erica, in turn, felt lonely and displaced. She had been a cheerleader and an honor-roll student in her small middle school, which she described as "like a family," and was finding it difficult to adjust to Jefferson's large size and aggressive atmosphere. Still, Erica struck me as a remarkably resilient and self-reliant adolescent. Her cousin, two years older, was the person to whom she was the closest and with whom she talked about sex. Together they were doing their best to resist the constant pressures from boys "to pop the cherry."

### Betsy Gordon and Cindy

Betsy Gordon was one of the first mothers to agree to be interviewed. She was determined that she and her daughters would have a more satisfying relationship than she had had with her own mother, and she hoped the project would help reopen the lines of communication with Cindy, fourteen, the younger of her two girls.

Both Betsy and her husband, Stan, reported a history of talking comfortably with their daughters about sex. They tried not to speak from a rigid point of view but instead to present as much information as they could, sharing their values and encouraging the girls to make their own decisions. This strategy had served them well in the past, but now, as Cindy was moving through adolescence, they were beginning to wonder if her independence and curiosity, once it became directed at sexuality, might lead her into trouble.

Cindy, a Nottingham eighth-grader with a strong will, clearly had been raised to think for herself, but now she was finding it harder to figure out what she wanted to do; new challenges were coming up that sometimes gave her pause. She showed a young adolescent's appreciation for her parents' support and openness. Still, she was discovering that boys were attracted to her and she to them, and she found it hard sometimes to talk openly with her parents. She didn't want to disappoint them.

### Joan Rankin and Carmen

The Rankins lived in a well-kept, modest house on a quiet city street near Jefferson. A trim fence with sprays of rose bushes gave the home an elegant touch, but there was nothing elaborate about their lifestyle. Joan, who had a master's degree in psychology, had recently lost her job at a small Catholic high school during budget cuts, and the family was struggling to make ends meet on her husband's salary from the city public works department. Two of their three children, fourteen-year-old Carmen and her younger brother, lived at home, while an older sister lived in her own apartment. Joan was hoping Carmen would get a fresh start at Jefferson.

Joan spoke about sex openly and frequently. She wanted Carmen to have correct factual information and, like Betsy Gordon, Evelyn Shepherd, and Mary Robbins, was able to answer Carmen's questions without too much discomfort. But as a convert to Catholicism, Joan also expected Carmen to follow the dictates of the Roman Catholic church.

Carmen was quiet and restrained and clearly had great respect for her parents. She felt the pressure to please them and to abide by their teachings and beliefs. At fourteen she had none of Cindy Gordon's confusion, because she believed she would be able to follow her parents' teachings and not, as Joan feared, "cave in to her environment."

### Gerry Valentia and Carolyn

Gerry Valentia's kitchen wasn't especially big, but it was the control center of her comfortable house in a working-class section of the city, and it was usually filled with teenagers passing through or hanging out. Among the four children, someone was always hungry or had hungry friends in tow. A serious chronic illness often sapped Gerry's stamina but not her sense of humor. She was the peacekeeper in the family and ran interference for the kids with their less flexible, more heavy-handed father.

Carolyn's two older siblings had been high achievers since nursery school, so when Carolyn failed to follow suit, her parents and teachers were caught by surprise. Academic difficulties were followed by social problems. Finally, after Carolyn and her mother had begun screaming at each other and Gerry was at her wits' end, they found an explanation: Carolyn was diagnosed with a learning disability. The school adjusted the curriculum and teaching methods to accommodate her learning style, and recently both her school performance and the atmosphere at home had improved. Also, she had become a rising star on Jefferson's basketball team, which had raised her self-confidence.

Gerry and Joe were Catholics, and their children had previously gone to Catholic schools, but the kids knew their mother believed that the church's teachings "should be taken with a few grains of salt." Fourteen-year-old Carolyn didn't hesitate to question anything that struck her as hypocritical or false, and this directness made for animated and sometimes tense family discussions.

### Phyllis Rosenbloom and Ruth

Conversations with Phyllis Rosenbloom often erupted into laughter. Phyllis was a darling, funny woman with a self-deprecating manner. If Ingrid Shepherd and her mother had the easiest and most open communication of the mothers and daughters I spoke with, Phyllis and Ruth, fifteen, had to be a close second. It was a surprise to Phyllis, then, when Ruth began talking less frequently and less openly with her. Phyllis wasn't sure what to make of her daughter's retreat. She'd been proud of their completely open relationship and was thrown for a loop by Ruth's increasing hesitancy and self-consciousness.

The Rosenblooms favored public school in theory, but with both parents working, Phyllis as a speech pathologist and Rick as a hospital administrator, they had moved their two girls to Nottingham for high school because of its extracurricular activities, scholastic emphasis, and small student-faculty ratio.

Ruth struck me as a serious young woman. Like her mother, she had a nice sense of humor, but she smiled less quickly and let questions percolate before deciding how to respond. Self-reflective, she seemed to have, for a fifteen-year-old, a mature grasp of both family and peer dynamics. She said that the girls she knew who were having sex weren't doing so because their biological drives were too strong to resist but because they thought it was expected of them.

### Marian Henderson and Tiffany

Like the Rosenblooms, the Hendersons, with fifteen-year-old Tiffany and two elementary-school-aged sons, lived in a suburb. Marian worked in the human resources department of a hospital, and her husband, Terrance, was an accounting supervisor with an insurance company. It had been a stretch financially to move Tiffany to Nottingham, but the Hendersons were unsatisfied with the local public school and, like the Rosenblooms, wanted their daughter's after-school hours filled constructively.

During Tiffany's early school years, Marian and Terrance had been separated for several years, and that period had fostered a special closeness between mother and daughter. When the Hendersons reconciled, Tiffany resented her father's return, and their relationship still had rough edges. When I met them, Tiffany was moving out of a rebellious phase and becoming more studious, but she was still holding back with her mom. While there was clearly great affection between mother and daughter, Tiffany was not yet ready to let her mother know when she agreed with her, and Marian was not sure just how much to trust her daughter's judgment.

### Emily Shattuck and Katrina

Many of the girls were mature for their age, but Katrina Shattuck seemed the most grown-up. Fifteen and coquettish, she easily could have convinced me she was nearing her college graduation. In fact, she was the family worrier and suffered severe periodic asthma attacks.

Though teased by her family about her penchant for worrying, she had legitimate anxieties. Her parents had divorced a few years earlier, and her mother had remarried. Since then, Katrina had chosen to live with her father, a high school principal, during the school year and spend school vacations and summers with her mother, stepfather, and seventeen-year-old sister. Both parents lived near Nottingham in comfortable homes, and the situation worked reasonably well. Still, Katrina felt guilty about not spending more time with her mom and often seemed to worry more about the adults in her family than the adults did about capable and responsible Katrina. Katrina's sister had recently become involved in a relationship with another young woman, which had sent the family into a tailspin. Katrina had become the self-appointed arbiter between her parents and her sister, but she felt torn about where to lend her support.

Emily had always had an open relationship with her daughters about sexual matters. They had talked about sexual activity, contraception, pregnancy, AIDS, abortion, and they agreed on every issue — except homosexuality. In the last three years, Emily had found raising her daughters more challenging than she had expected, with easy communication much less frequent, and she was frustrated. With her daughters' not confiding in her as readily as they once had, Emily sometimes found herself eavesdropping or reading their letters to discover what was going on in their lives.

### Alma Parks and Angela

"Pistol" is the word to describe fifteen-year-old Angela Parks. About five foot four inches tall, she exuded a don't-mess-with-me air that gave her an imposing presence. When she came into the room, she took possession of it. It was no surprise to learn that the Jefferson faculty considered her an outstanding student leader and that she had been part of many city-wide and national activities for remarkable students. Among her peers she was a promoter of better understanding of African-American achievements.

Angela's mother was enormously proud of her oldest daughter's confidence and academic success. Alma had come to her own independence slowly: after a teenage pregnancy and an unhappy marriage that produced four children, she had only recently decided to try life on her own. She'd left the South, moved her children to a small duplex in the city, taken two jobs, and enrolled in college. Her favorite theme was the importance of education, which she stressed constantly with her children. She did not want them diverted by sex, which she told Angela was "a drug that once you try it, you become addicted."

### Dorothy Dodson and Anita
### Diane Early and Melinda

Anita Dodson and Melinda Early were both fifteen, freshmen at Jefferson living with divorced mothers and in relatively stable, sexually active relationships with young men. Though not social friends, they spoke about their relationships in similar ways. Each one felt she and her boyfriend had approached the subject of sex slowly and cautiously, taking time to test their feelings and discuss the implications of their actions. Both girls took care to use contraceptives, and both reported feeling comfortable with the decisions they had made, even if sometimes there seemed to be deeper feelings etched beneath their words. Melinda was concerned that her mother and grandmother would find out about her relationship; knowing that they would disapprove, she felt apprehensive and was avoiding her grandmother. Anita's uneasiness, on the other hand, was related to the rape she had experienced at age eleven and the effects of that traumatic event on her current relationship.

Physically and temperamentally, the two girls couldn't have been more different. Anita was carefully groomed, curvaceous, and classically pretty. She had a soft voice and a sexy aura about her. Melinda, on the other hand, was tall, large-boned, and loudly outspoken. During our counseling sessions at Jefferson, Melinda would amuse the girls with the boldest questions, the most outrageous comments, and the rudest quips.

Anita had recently left a much more secure life in Florida. She and her four siblings, along with her mother and father, had lived in a safe suburban neighborhood. Her father had run a successful contracting business and the family had enjoyed a comfortable middle-class life — until Dewayne Dodson asked his wife of twenty years for a divorce. A dad who had been involved in his children's lives, he was missed for his presence as well as the economic security he had assured. Dorothy had come with four of the children to a third-floor walk-up in one of the city's rougher blue-collar neighborhoods, and in the short time they had been there, Anita had already faced a near-rape situation.

Dorothy appeared tired and still stunned by the curveball life had thrown her. She was job hunting, but with two children in elementary school, it was hard to find work that gave her the flexibility she needed. She described Anita as "a real day-brightener of a child."

By comparison, Melinda's life seemed easier. Her mother worked in the records department of a large company, and they lived in an attractive duplex on a quiet street. Melinda and her mother considered themselves very close emotionally, and Melinda said they were able to discuss anything — except sex. The topic had become uncomfortable when Melinda was almost twelve and Diane had ended a long-term relationship, married another man, borne a son, and divorced. The boy, now four and the focus of the household, ensured that there were few quiet times in the house. Melinda knew that her mother was again involved with her former boyfriend, but it was hardly discussed. Now that Melinda had become sexually active, she turned more to her aunt for information.

### Pauline Dickinson and Tina Watts

Although two years older than Cindy and Ingrid, Tina, at sixteen seemed much younger. She had experienced years of physical and sexual abuse from a stepfather and, in her teens, had been taken from her mother's home and placed with her great-aunt, Pauline. Tina was trying to heed her aunt's advice, but she missed her mother and sister and daydreamed about returning home.

Pauline Dickinson, a sixty-year-old retired child care worker, had been widowed early and had successfully raised four children on her own. Her eighth-grade education was supplemented by a lifetime of observation about how parents and children interacted. A wise, grand-motherly woman, she understood Tina's wounds and was working hard to raise her with kindness and care. Pauline had encouraged her niece to go to weekly confession and church services and arranged for her to meet regularly with a counselor, but Tina remained enormously vul-nerable.

Tina was becoming more interested in boys, and Pauline learned that she had skipped school one day to spend the afternoon with a boy. When Pauline asked Tina if they had had sexual intercourse, Tina said yes. The boy, she explained, wanted her to do it and would have gotten mad if she hadn't. Pauline kept a hawk's eye on Tina after that incident, talking with her frequently about being responsible and mak-ing her own decisions, but the scars of Tina's childhood remained raw. Starved for affection, Tina was thinking, even at her young age, about getting married and having children.

### Estelle Brown and Samantha

Sitting in Estelle Brown's living room, sipping coffee, and talking was a calming experience. Harold Brown was a well-recognized medical scholar, and the elegant home of this family, close to Nottingham, was lined with books and art. Estelle was an active community volunteer. Although sophisticated and at ease in many social circles, she was temperamentally reserved and private. Both she and her husband had difficulty discussing sexual topics during Sam's adolescence.

Instead it was Aunt Dee, her mother's sister in Oklahoma, to whom Samantha turned with her most private questions and confusing thoughts. Many nights, after finishing her homework, Sam would curl up in bed and chat long distance with her aunt at length. Estelle had encouraged this family connectedness, but at the time we were meeting, Estelle had begun to feel uneasy that she hadn't contributed enough to her daughter's sexual education. Seeing her mature and attractive seventeen-year-old daughter becoming a woman, she had made a point to try and "set the stage" for conversation. Like so many of the mother-daughter pairs, Sam and Estelle were attempting the high-wire act of getting the conversation about sex right without its being an enormously uncomfortable — or counterproductive — experience.

These fifteen mother-daughter pairs speak to the situations of many families in our society today. Eight of the girls were living in single-parent families with a mother or aunt, either because of divorce or because an aunt had assumed a guardian role. Factors such as the mother's education, economic stability, and the ongoing involvement of each girl's father affected the relationship between mother and daughter — and thus their communication about sexual issues. Single moms especially were well aware of the hardships and pain that an unwanted pregnancy could bring to their daughters' lives and to their own. Those with higher educational levels, such as Cybil Mason and Mary Robbins, may have been able to articulate some of their concerns to their daughters with careful arguments; however, those with less formal education, such as Alma Parks and Pauline Dickinson, had learned through life's experiences the jeopardy of early sexual entanglement. At times, the direct communication that seemed to be more common in single-parent homes led to more open and heated arguments, but these fights did not diminish the emotional connectedness in the mother-daughter relationship — and at times even may have worked to strengthen it.

On the other hand, in the seven two-parent households, mothers exhibited less frustration and feelings of isolation in their efforts to talk with daughters about sexual issues. Though most of the fathers were not directly involved in their adolescent daughters' lives, these mothers could turn to their husbands for backup. They could share problems and work together on some of the issues that inevitably arose with their adolescents. That is not to say that the emotional relationship between mother and daughter in these households was any stronger than in single-parent homes, but mothers in two-parent families generally had more financial and emotional support to draw on in coping with their daughters' concerns.

The key difference I found between these familial situations was that single mothers talked more directly with daughters about protecting themselves from physical and emotional harm than mothers in two-parent homes. The experiences some of the single mothers had had in their own lives, especially dating interactions, made them sensitive to their daughters' vulnerabilities, and they hammered their points home.

Though fathers didn't often come up in our conversations, they could and did help their daughters in indirect ways as the girls struggled to sort through their relationships with boys and peers. While it was obviously easier for fathers living in the same household to be available and interact with their daughters frequently, some of the divorced fathers were also working to stay involved.

In addition, cultural values and practices seemed to play a role in the way that these girls were learning about sex and sexuality. Several of the African-American mother-daughter pairs I met with, for instance, spoke of how their families encouraged teenage girls to talk with female relatives about sex and other adolescent concerns. Grandmothers, great-aunts, and aunts were all invaluable fonts of information and support. One mother described a tradition in her own family: "My mother, my grandmother, my great-aunts, and all the old ladies would sit about and talk. . . . You could graduate from one level to the other. There was one point when you were very young . . . you weren't even allowed to get into the room with them, as they're talking about these things that they would consider SEX. Then . . . as you got older, they would allow you to sit in the room but not talk. . . . If you chose to open your mouth, then you would have to leave because you weren't really mature enough to *add* to the conversation. . . . Finally you would get to the point where you really felt that you'd made it if you had actually contributed something to the conversation. So I learned from them." Mothers who had familial backup for their daughters appeared to breathe a bit easier, knowing that if they failed to communicate something important, a family member would come to the rescue.[2]

All of the mothers and daughters I interviewed, but especially these fifteen, are collaborators in this project. Their wide range of experiences details in full color both the difficulties and the rewards of communication between mothers and daughters.

# THREE

# From Little Girl
# to Young Venus

## NURTURING GIRLS
## THROUGH ADOLESCENCE

❧

Just before my daughter was to turn eleven, our family moved from Newton, Massachusetts, to Galveston, Texas. This meant that Katherine would start sixth grade in a large, diverse middle school rather than in our small, familiar neighborhood elementary school. When we drove up to her new school the first day, I was struck by how adult the students appeared. I remember thinking that *all* of the girls seemed very mature physically — certainly much more so than my petite eleven-year-old daughter, who was wearing her favorite bell-bottom jeans and earth shoes.

During those first few weeks, Katherine cried almost every morning, begging not to go to school and sometimes even throwing up. We met with her counselors and the principal to find ways to support her and help her feel more comfortable. She talked about the scariness of going from class to class and her fears that she wouldn't find the right room before the bell rang and that she might have to go to the bathroom and be late to class. For a few days I walked the halls between periods disguised in sunglasses and a bandanna, shadowing Katherine as she gratefully moved among the older children without ever acknowledging my presence.

Slowly things got better for her in her new school. The earth shoes and bell-bottoms were thrown to the back of the closet, and my daughter's clothing began to mimic that of the more mature girls. But as Katherine became happier, I found myself oddly sad. I was glad, certainly, that she was adjusting to her new school and beginning to feel more comfortable, but these events, which seemed to foreshadow the end of Katherine's childhood, left me with a bittersweet feeling. When the mother of a fourteen-year-old at Jefferson told me, "I still see the little girl there, and to think about her becoming a sexual being . . . it's just weird. In a way she's still this grubby little kid. She doesn't even bathe half the time if I don't tell her. . . . She still plays with toys some of the time. And to see it coming . . ." She trailed off. I knew just how she felt.

The feeling that our girls are suddenly growing up too quickly and too soon is one that several of the moms mentioned. Mary Robbins, for instance, noted Vicki was just "getting into puberty" at age thirteen, though "all her friends have been there for maybe a year or two longer. She still has a child's figure even though she's five foot six." As with many middle-school girls, Vicki was bouncing back and forth between childhood fascinations and preadolescent behavior. "If you put her in with a bunch of ten-, eleven-, or twelve-year-olds, she fits in beautifully," explained her mom. "If they're playing dolls, she's right there with the doll play. And twenty minutes later, if the room changed and she were with all teenagers, she'd be right there with them, too."

This vacillation between old interests and new teen passions can be understandably disconcerting for moms. How are we supposed to know whether to talk with them about dolls or rock groups? And, if we treasured our close relationship with our little girls, it can be all the more difficult to see them start to befriend older teens, watch as their wardrobes undergo a radical transformation, or listen as their sentences become dotted with "like." Rest assured, however, that this is the natural course of girls trying on adolescence, as mothers described it time and again.

## Between Dolls and Lip Gloss

The common experience of watching adolescent daughters swing from cuddly to capricious can make two women fast friends. That kind of camaraderie blossomed when Mary Robbins and I first met over the phone. Mary was eager for mother-talk. On the day of our interview, I waited in a sleek conference room until an elegant woman in a pink designer suit and neat chignon appeared in the doorway. She dazzled me with a beautiful smile, even more striking against her warm brown skin.

Mary had become a mother at thirty-three. Just a few years later her marriage dissolved, but Vicki's father remained a committed and involved parent. Mary spoke warmly of all the good times she and Vicki had shared, but she noted the crazy juggling act of balancing the demands of a busy career and an energetic thirteen-year-old.

Beyond Vicki's fluctuating childhood interests and teenage passions, Mary was just beginning to notice with Vicki the "testing" that many young adolescent girls engage in. "She has some pretty profound ideas that I've always found surprising," Mary began. "She has an ability to look closely into things and come up with an understanding that you would never expect of someone that age." But with Vicki's clear thinking came a strong will that presented parental challenges. "Vicki will try to be in charge," Mary explained. "Sometimes I'm so tired I let her get away with some of it; other times I say, 'This is just totally unacceptable.' I have to tell her that I happen to be the mother and I know that it's done this way."

Struggling to be a good disciplinarian without squashing Vicki's spirited nature, Mary tried to set realistic limits. Vicki was encouraged to bring up any subject she wanted and was free to disagree with her parents, so long as she did so with respect and a willingness to sit down and talk. Vicki later told me this approach made her feel grownup, but she confessed that having a temper tantrum sometimes also "felt good" and got her what she wanted. When I asked if she and her mom argued, she responded nonchalantly, "Oh, sure, but mostly we fight over stupid stuff, like the time I tried to tell her it was her job to clean out the turtle cage because she was the mother."

For the time being, Mary's main concerns for Vicki fell squarely on offering guidance without being overbearing. She alluded, though, to the challenges ahead. Vicki's headstrong qualities signaled her emerging adolescence, and Mary anticipated the physical changes that awaited her daughter. Right now Vicki was tall and slightly overweight, and Mary worried that Vicki's verbal acuity might cause people to forget that her emotions were still those of a young girl. "You see how big she is at thirteen. . . . I worry," she said. "You see so many girls who are overweight, and finally somebody looks at them twice. Instead of being careful, it's just like they're totally in love because someone paid attention to them."

Despite the obstacles ahead, Mary looked forward to watching her daughter evolve into a young woman. Their close relationship, she hoped, would carry them through whatever hormonal firestorms puberty had in store. Though we shared the inevitable sadness that comes with the end of the little-girl years, Mary concluded, "I'm curious to see who she'll be as an adult and how she'll get there."

## The Precariousness of Confidence

When I first met Vicki Robbins, she had the fresh confidence and charm of a young girl. Her oversized blouse hung loosely outside her full, short skirt, and she was wonderfully unselfconscious in the way she carried herself. Despite the wariness her mother had expressed earlier, Vicki's expression didn't appear to be inhibited by her weight or size. She shared Mary's generous smile and spoke with assurance. When I asked her what came to mind when she thought about being a teenager, she immediately said, "The first thing that comes to mind is *boys*. I notice them differently than I used to. Before I just looked at them and thought, Oh, he's nice. Okay. But now I look at a boy and think, What a nice build." She added, "I think more about his personality, his attitude about things and what he thinks of me. I notice that lots of boys my age are immature, and so I like the boys who are older than me — not too much, like about seventeen."

Having said her piece on boys, she talked with pride about her relationship with both her mom and her dad and her confidence that they would always be available to help her work through tough decisions. Her grandparents were taking her on a vacation shortly, and she basked in the warmth and support of her mother's extended family. Without hesitation, Vicki expressed her firm opinions to me.

Yet despite her quest for mature boys, she also held on to some girlhood interests. She recently had been lobbying for a new computer game from her mom, since Nintendo had been outlawed in their home. She confided her strategy: "I tell my mom, 'Oh, you look gorgeous today.'" She added, "I've been loving her and hugging her. . . . I've been working hard for that Gameboy." Mischievousness aside, she quickly added, "I really do love my mother."

Like any mom, I was moved by this admission, but Vicki soon reminded me I was dealing with a canny adolescent. "After we finish the interview," she asked, "would you go in and tell my mother that it makes kids happy when they can have Gameboy?" Suddenly I was her newfound conspirator. "It won't hurt. You can tell her that and she'll never know that I told you." At thirteen, Vicki was vivacious, eager to have fun, and confident.

My next interview, with Bettina Mason, a few days shy of fourteen, was a study in contrasts. If Vicki was exuberant, Bettina was skittish and reticent. When I arrived at the Mason home in a leafy suburb, Cybil greeted me warmly and talked in an easy, open manner. Like Mary Robbins, Cybil had been divorced for a decade, but she didn't have the same supportive family relationships. With a mother both she and Bettina found difficult and judgmental and sisters who were battling depression, Cybil longed for a healthy, happy home life for her daughter. As we talked, I noticed Bettina's portrait on the living room wall. She was an attractive young girl with blond hair, pale skin, and blue eyes.

Her mom described Bettina as a very good student, "one who sets her own goals and goes for them." What's more, she was an excellent writer: "her teachers have said she writes like a senior in high school." Bettina, according to Cybil, was "very perceptive about people and relationships and has a great sense of humor." Everything in her mom's description suggested that here was a young teen ready to take the world by storm.

But when Bettina entered the living room for our meeting, saying goodbye to her mom, she gave me a quick "Hello" with a slight smile. Her eyes remained fixed on the carpet while she arranged herself carefully in her chair. She gingerly put her hands in her lap and crossed her legs at the ankles. To begin our conversation, I shared a story about interviewing a girl who had asked me, "Do you want to know what I think or do you want to know what I *really* think?" Bettina smiled. I told her I hoped she would feel comfortable telling me what she *really* thought. This didn't seem to spur her on; she was obviously waiting for prompting. When I asked what was the first thing that came to mind about being a teenage girl, rather than launching into a whirlwind description as Vicki had, Bettina responded, still not looking at me, "I don't know. What do you mean?"

"Anything you think," I told her.

"It's good . . . I guess," she said. "I like being older, and um . . . oh . . . I don't know." She continued, "I like being independent. . . . I don't like to rely on my parents as much . . . like when I go down the street to visit a friend, I don't have to have my mother with me." As she spoke, she kept pulling out phrases of uncertainty, such as "I guess," "I'm like, um," and "I don't know." Later, when analyzing the transcript of our interview, I counted forty-five "I don't know"s with almost as many "I guess"s and "Like, I mean"s sprinkled into her answers. Even when Bettina ventured saying something straight out, such as, "I think I should know about ways to prevent diseases and stuff when you have sex," she would qualify it with "Well, I'm really not sure" or "I don't know." Ambivalence seemed to be her currency.

Here was a bright young adolescent who was quite accomplished but who conveyed little self-confidence or curiosity in our meeting. What was she really thinking? Was she simply shy or hesitant with me, or was something else going on?

Given Vicki and Bettina's similar ages and their shared track record of accolades, the differences in how they conducted themselves in conversation were striking. Vicki had been bursting to talk about what was on her mind and appeared to have fun in the process. Bettina, I felt, was more concerned with answering my questions correctly. And when she was uncertain what would be "correct," she avoided answering altogether. What was going on here?

According to a report by the American Association of University Women (AAUW), the number of girls who strongly agree with the phrase "I like most things about myself" drops thirteen points between elementary and middle school and one additional point between middle school and high school. Clearly a change takes hold of many girls in early adolescence. As some of the feminist researchers who have studied teenagers have described, these girls often place such a high value on their responses to other people's needs and requests that their self-interest can travel virtually "underground."[1] Some are experiencing new changes in their bodies as well. Bettina, for instance, was beginning to show signs of a young woman's physical development, while Vicki still had a young girl's body.

My conversations with Vicki and Bettina and the other girls highlighted early on not just the ways in which they were talking about boys and sexuality but also the broader issues of how they were confronting the world and how, though perhaps close in age, they brought remarkably different levels of poise and self-assurance to our conversations — and, for that matter, to the whole business of adolescence. Some were approaching it with gusto, others with uncertainty.

Such differences, as I began to see in speaking with mother-daughter pairs, are critical to keep in mind as we nurture each teenager through adolescence and as we determine effective communication strategies. What might be an easy conversation about adolescent topics with one girl could be incredibly difficult with another. And, if a girl's self-confidence drops during the junior high years, how will she tackle the more daunting dilemmas of adolescence? How can we expect her, for instance, to be comfortable with her emerging sexuality in her adolescent relationships if she doesn't first feel confident about herself in school, in her extracurricular activities, and at home?

It is this background that we need in order to consider the confusion of sexuality for an adolescent girl.

## A Brief History of Adolescent Development

Looking back on the history of developmental psychological theory, we can see that we have come a long way in understanding how girls progress through adolescence. Until the 1970s, academics thought they had an accurate theoretical grasp of how young people like Vicki and Bettina moved into adulthood. In the 1960s Erik Erikson, expanding on Freud's theories, developed the psychosocial stages of human development and devised the now well known theory that a child must take certain steps to become a healthy adult. Erikson further explained that children must separate from their parents in order to establish their own identity.[2]

According to Erikson, children pass through five stages before arriving at adulthood.[3] Fast-forwarding to the fifth stage brings us to adolescence — a stage that some mothers might well compare to crossing a deep, swirling river. Erikson explained that during this critical period in maturation a teen begins to develop an independent identity. Faced with a physiological revolution within and with adult tasks ahead, adolescents become focused on their image in the eyes of others as compared with their own self-image. Erikson defined the adolescent mind as "essentially a mind of the moratorium" between childhood and adulthood, between the morality learned by the child and the ethics to be developed by the adult. It is in this stage that the external affirmation of peers and the rituals, creeds, and programs of the community are especially influential on development.

These important theories were used to make sense of both boys' and girls' development, but as it happened, Erikson, like previous researchers, did not go far enough. Their theories were based almost exclusively on male models of behavior. Though it may be hard to believe today, no one at the time had thought to look closely at whether young girls matured differently from boys. When girls did not follow the given models, instead of questioning the theories, psychologists and psychiatrists developed explanations to account for female "deficiencies."[4]

Given how much we have come to understand in recent years, it may be hard to appreciate the originality of the work of people like Carol Gilligan, Nancy Chodorow, and Jean Baker Miller, who in the 1970s and 1980s began looking specifically at girls and documenting the ways their development consistently diverged from that of boys.[5] When Gilligan's book on female development, *In a Different Voice*, appeared in 1982, thousands of women around the country responded with an enormous *Yes!* Finally, here was a book explaining with academic research what we already knew in our hearts — that boys and girls develop their own identity in different ways. Where others had negatively characterized nonconforming female behavior with such terms as "dependent," "immature," or "inferior," Gilligan saw it as simply different. Gilligan and other feminist researchers shed dramatic new light on girls' development, demonstrating the importance of relationships and the high influence of culture on girls. Also, they showed that many girls begin to move into uncertainty about what they think and how they feel as they enter adolescence.

Many of my conversations with mothers and daughters confirmed the findings of these previous women researchers. Every girl develops differently and reaches puberty at her own speed. But, for the most part, girls on the edge of adolescence, like Vicki, were usually confident and spunky in our conversations. Outspoken about their thoughts and feelings, most of the younger girls discussed relationships freely with me. They talked about how close they felt to family members and, in particular, to their mothers. Those daughters who were deeper into adolescence, both physically and emotionally, however, sometimes seemed confused, unsure, and reticent to speak about their views. Clarity and outspokenness had given way to those commonplace phrases "I don't know" and "I'm not sure." Earlier research found that through early adolescence girls usually continue to be energetic, assertive, and outspoken, as Vicki demonstrated with fanfare. But self-confidence can easily be eroded as girls move further into puberty. How is this relevant to nurturing our daughters through their teens, especially concerning understanding sexuality?

Bettina's mother appeared to be skillful in talking with her about sexual issues and supportive of her academic and other interests. Cybil spoke of wanting to make sure Bettina recognized that a good relationship is one in which two people work together and neither one dominates or manipulates the other. Yet Bettina seemed to be picking up other messages from her environment as well, talking with concern, for instance, about her aunts' depression and her grandmother's critical eye. And with her parents' divorce in the background, she knew that life wasn't always easy. The messages that are pervasive in our culture about "appropriate" behavior for teenage girls seemed to have futherr contributed to Bettina's hesitancy in our interview.

From their research at a private girls' school in Ohio, Lynn Brown and Carol Gilligan determined that adolescent girls were silenced not by internal developmental processes but by the socialization they experienced. Pat Flanders Hall, an administrator at the school, reflected on what they heard from the girls. "We listened to the voices of the girls tell us that it was the adult women in their lives that provided models for silencing themselves and behaving like 'good little girls.'" Listening to the girls, Hall said, "we wept," and concluded that "unless we, as grown women, were willing to give up all the 'good little girl' things we continued to do and give up our expectation that the girls in our charge would be as good as we were, we could not successfully empower young women to act on their own knowledge and feelings. Unless we stopped hiding in expectations of goodness and control, our behavior would silence any words to girls about speaking in their own voice."[6]

These are important words for mothers to heed. That isn't to say that we can make sweeping assumptions that for every girl a move toward timidity in adolescence signals the lack of strong female role models or vice versa. But what Brown and Gilligan's work does point to is the need for greater awareness of the obstacles that adolescent girls are confronting as they develop an independent identity and the fact that they look to mothers for guidance. If girls struggle to find confident voices on the most basic of issues in early adolescence, it is all the more important that we provide them a comfortable space to speak out about sexuality, to let them know it is okay to feel confused or to want to ask questions.

All but one of the young adolescent girls I spoke with named their mothers as the prime purveyor of information when it came to sexual matters. Jenny King, at thirteen, gushed with admiration for her mom: "She's funny and she laughs a lot . . . and she lets me wear her clothes." When it came to talking about sex, Jenny reported, "I can ask her about anything. I'll go up and ask her about masturbation . . . and that'll sort of start a conversation."

As our daughters begin to explore their body changes and ideas about sex and sexuality, mothers can provide invaluable role models. Girls are looking to mothers not only for larger life lessons but also for information and guidance on matters of puberty and sexuality. Because mothers and daughters share an indivisible bond, what we say about the issues of womanhood has great potential to resonate with our girls.

## Edging Toward Maturity

If our daughters' sudden interest in dress and makeup seems at odds with their continuing girlhood passions, if their confidence seems to go underground for a period, even more startling may be the disjunction between physical development and emotional maturity. Making sure that we're addressing the right part of the equation can be a mind-boggling task.

For most girls, changes such as breast development, the growth of underarm and pubic hair, and the development of the uterus and vagina, usually occur over two to three years. Yet for both moms and girls it can feel as if such changes happen overnight. In the months after our first meeting, Vicki, though still girlishly chubby, shot up in height and began menstruating. Though Bettina had begun menstruating at age twelve, her body developed more curves, with small breasts and rounded hips.

As one mother of a twelve-year-old confided, "She has a woman's body and a child's mind, and I'm worried." Another mom aptly compared the passage through puberty to an orchestra of talented musicians in which the strings are playing at one speed, the drums are beating, much faster, and the horns are sounding with slow elegance: some dissonance is inevitable.

When Karen walked into my office at Jefferson wanting to talk about her new life as a high school student, I was surprised to learn that she was only fourteen. Her tall, willowy figure, stylish brown hair, and well-manicured nails suggested a much older young woman. In fact, Karen said that most of her friends were seventeen or eighteen. But as her story unfolded, it became clear that her emotional maturity was not in sync with her physical development and that she was still interested in girlhood pastimes.

This cool and sophisticated young woman revealed how frightened she really was about becoming a teenager. Having watched several of her older friends become pregnant and drop out of school, Karen wondered how she could possibly avoid their mistakes. As a young girl she had had to take on enormous responsibilities; when she was just eleven, her mother's drug habit escalated, leaving Karen with the adult responsibility of caring for herself and her younger brothers.

But when the conversation turned to her interests, she animatedly talked about her porcelain doll collection. She described her dolls in loving detail and identified them by name. "That's the only thing I'm interested in," she said. "I'm always going to collect them." Underneath her brave and polished exterior, Karen was very much a little girl, deeply lonely and in search of guidance. Her dolls provided her with a safe touchstone.

So often the seemingly abrupt physical changes of adolescence make girls, not to mention parents, anxious, especially when they occur earlier than usual.[7] Instead of enjoying the emergence of womanly characteristics, girls may become overwhelmed and confused. There is also evidence that girls who move into puberty early may be especially vulnerable to peer pressure and diminished self-esteem. When a young adolescent experiences the rapid development of primary and secondary sexual characteristics such as breasts, hips, and pubic hair, she quickly has to acquire new perceptions of her body. All adolescents feel some anxiety as they progress through puberty, but for the early bloomers, the anxiety and feelings of inadequacy or inferiority may be more pronounced. These stresses may also result in variable school performance, eating disorders, or other anxieties.

Girls, like Karen, who look much older physically may become involved with older, more experienced adolescents because they *look* as though they belong with this group. And spending time with older teens may lead a girl who is still emotionally and intellectually immature to follow their behaviors in hopes of being accepted by that peer group.

It becomes doubly important, then, for parents to respond to these early bloomers in terms of their intellectual and emotional rather than physical development. Though they may look — and act — like young women, the odds are they are not yet ready to take on the separation issues of midadolescence. They still need parental hugs. A structured schedule that keeps their energies focused on activities with others who match their emotional development, rather than hanging out with older boys and girls, can help physically mature young teens stay the course.

## Starting Conversation Early

The good news is that at least until girls begin puberty, mothers are an easily accessible and influential resource for them about body changes and sexual issues. Most mothers and daughters reported that they had had discussions about puberty and menarche before girls began menstruating and that these conversations had been positive. Even those mothers who hadn't had the most open of relationships with their daughters were pleasantly surprised to discover that the onset of menstruation provided an ideal time to bolster communication around issues of sex and sexuality. At this moment the daughter has tangible proof that she is maturing, entering her mother's world. It's a good time for conversations about sex, relationships, trust, and judgment.

Although they may not be ready to process all the information that mothers want to impart, younger girls are generally open to conversations about the nuts and bolts of reproduction and puberty. And if moms have signaled a willingness to respond to questions, girls will frequently ask them without much embarrassment. Because their questions typically pertain to such general topics as conception, body changes, and menstruation, the majority of mothers I spoke with felt comfortable and reasonably knowledgeable providing the answers.

Even when questions become more advanced or detailed, mothers of girls in middle school perceive the questions to be general information-gathering. They are not yet concerned that answering a question about sex will be misconstrued as condoning sexual activity, and daughters have not yet begun to worry about what their moms might think of them for asking.

Some of the younger girls I spoke with reported that they had not given much thought to becoming sexually active and weren't all that interested in discussing it. As one seventh-grader at Nottingham summed up: "I really don't want to know anything. I just want to go on with life and not have to worry about that. Okay?" Their attitude was that they would learn only what they needed to know at this stage.

Their mothers echoed that view. Developmentally, the girls were "just not there yet." The mothers didn't consider it appropriate to discuss in detail matters of pregnancy, birth control, and premarital sex with their young adolescent girls, who were just becoming interested in boys and hadn't begun dating yet.

Ingrid Shepherd, at fourteen, had recently moved into midadolescence, however, and she was beginning to show interest in sexual issues well beyond the mechanics of reproduction. Ingrid and her mother, Evelyn, were by far the best communicators I encountered, and their open relationship no doubt contributed to the easiness with which Ingrid broached some of the broader issues of sex and sexuality.

An early bloomer physically, Ingrid also was well poised emotionally to ask her mother more detailed questions.

One day Ingrid was perusing the tabloids while her mom waited in the checkout line at the grocery store. She spied the headline BOY CASTRATES SELF. "So," Ingrid recalled, "I yell across to my mom, 'Mom, what does "castrate" mean?' There's like this dead hush, and everyone is looking at my mom to see what she is going to say. My mom laughs and motions me close," Ingrid recounted. " 'Ingrid, do you know the difference between a gelding and a stallion?' She knows I've been around horses a lot and I've watched a lot of nature specials. 'That's what it means.' " In telling this story, Ingrid displayed pride in her mother's openness. Here was a girl who was learning that curiosity and conversation didn't get her into trouble and that her voice could be heard, even in public, even on sexual issues.

Evelyn and her husband had begun to prepare Ingrid for the changes in her body at an early age. When Ingrid started getting breasts at age eight, Evelyn bought her a bra and also seized the opportunity to talk about menstruation. Ingrid recalled, "My parents sat down with me with this big book [about reproduction]. It was like a picture book. They showed me pictures and explained what they meant. My dad sat next to me. He was flipping through and explaining things." Suddenly it dawned on her: "My dad does this!" At first she was taken aback, as most children are when they think about their parents engaging in sex. But then, she said, she thought about it and figured, "Well, why not; parents are people too."

If young people have trouble comprehending that their parents are sexual beings, parents face a similar reality check. It can be hard to fathom that a daughter who still seems so much the little girl is ready to receive detailed sexual information. Yet in my conversations with girls, two things became clear. First, they generally will not receive or will not retain information they are not ready for. Either they will say, "No, I don't want to hear about that," or they will let the information fall away. Second, mothers who postpone discussing the basics of sex and sexual development until they think their daughters are "mature enough" may find they have misjudged the time when daughters are most likely to engage in easy conversation.

Ingrid confided that talking with her parents about sex felt strange at times, even embarrassing. "I was little bit uncomfortable," she recalled. "But then I thought back, and I thought, We've been talking about this stuff for a long time and just because I'm changing doesn't mean that communication has to stop. You hear a lot about teenagers not talking to their parents. I think that's really stupid."

By talking early, often, and easily with Ingrid, Evelyn Shepherd increased the odds of communicating successfully with her daughter through adolescence.[8] They had established a comfort level for discussing sexual topics and were armed with successful ways of talking that would help them in those inevitable difficult moments ahead. If Ingrid did retreat later, she would already have a reservoir of useful information.

Not all mothers are as comfortable discussing sexuality as Evelyn Shepherd, nor are all daughters as outspoken and assertive as Ingrid. It isn't important to be able to explain castration in the supermarket line without blushing. What is critical is that we assure our daughters early on and into midadolescence that puberty and sex are reasonable topics for inquiry just as much as cooking, sports, or math and that even if a question cannot be answered readily, that does not mean it is inappropriate.

## When Daughters Pull Away: Strategies That Work – and That Don't

Both Ingrid and Evelyn anticipated some difficult moments ahead. As Evelyn put it, "Who knows what is going to happen when the hormones kick in at age sixteen and she falls madly in love?" The other mothers and daughters I spoke with confirmed that once they got past the emotional and physical disjunctions of early adolescence and menarche, other challenges, including girls' hormone surges, invariably arose. Most mothers agreed that somewhere between the ages of thirteen and sixteen, girls underwent a sea change (some witnessed it as early as age twelve). Suddenly conflicts escalated and daughters, instead of being eager to comply with their mothers' wishes, became disagreeable and somewhat aloof.

In midadolescence, girls are in the process of drawing boundaries between themselves and their mothers, with whom they have been most closely affiliated during childhood. Part of shaping their own identity, figuring out who they want to become in this new thing called womanhood, means testing — not just themselves but those around them.[9] Bedrooms often become a point of contention. Many teenage girls become slobs, and their mothers hate it.

In addition, girls' concerns about sexual issues seem to become more personal and pointed. At fifteen, Tiffany Henderson, just moving out of her rebellious phase, described her sudden newfound interest in sex: "I started learning about it [sexual activity] in seventh grade, but I never realized — it didn't sort of mean anything to me until about last year. About fourteen. Because, like, I never even thought about it. I just thought I grew up and started, you know, thinking about boys more."

As girls approach midadolescence, their self-image becomes increasingly associated with how they perceive their bodies and how others, particularly boys, perceive them. Suddenly they begin to think of themselves as sexual beings. They become increasingly curious about sexual activity — who's doing it and with whom — and how their peers' behaviors may influence how they themselves act in a dating situation. They're walking a tightrope: they want to be viewed by boys as sexually attractive, but they also are uncertain who they will be as teenagers.

As their curiosity escalates, so too does their ambivalence about what questions to ask and concerns to share with their mothers. They want their moms to hold them in high esteem, and suddenly it feels as if broaching these topics might jeopardize their mothers' golden regard. Likewise, mothers begin to detect vibes that their girls are taking a more sexual interest in boys. The switch can catch a parent off guard, and conversations can become embarrassing. As one ninth-grader put it, "I think it's just being embarrassed, you know, that like this is my mom and she's old, and she never did any of this."

Even if daughters and mothers can overcome their mutual embarrassment, some mothers feel that bringing up some of these topics might encourage a daughter's heightened interest in sexual activity. This thought sends many on a fast retreat — so they don't say anything at all. Midadolescence is often a difficult stage, with issues that have seemingly higher stakes, and getting through it usually requires different communication tactics from those that worked during early adolescence. A mother may try to initiate discussion about a sexual topic, only to have her daughter leave the room or turn away with a remark like "I know that already." At this stage the old saying "Patience is a virtue" takes on new meaning.

Ruth Rosenbloom and her mother, Phyllis, had an easygoing relationship much like Ingrid and Evelyn Shepherd's — until Ruth turned fifteen. From grade school through middle school, Ruth and her older sister had inundated Phyllis with questions about oral sex, masturbation, sexually transmitted diseases, and any other question that came to mind. Phyllis, in turn, strove to respond as best she could. But in Ruth's fifteenth year, mother and daughter were communicating less directly and less comfortably. Ruth had become a young woman, physically and intellectually. She now thought she could easily calculate the consequences of various behaviors without consulting her mother.

But along with Ruth's newfound maturity, her mother witnessed a withdrawal from family conversations. Phyllis said she thought Ruth was more confident when she was younger. "It started in seventh grade," Phyllis explained. "She went from being this confident [girl] to being more unsure . . . I really don't know what happened."

Ruth was beginning to realize that her interest in sexual issues had become more personal, and this made her reluctant to broach topics with her mom. Suddenly, asking for sexual information felt awkward. "Now I don't always answer all my mom's questions," she said. "I don't know, it just doesn't seem mother-daughter–like. Even if I said what I am thinking to my mom, she wouldn't be shocked or anything like that. I think she'd probably want me to say [what I'm thinking] to her. But it just seems to me that maybe I'd feel weird about things, or I'd be worried that she'd look at me differently." With a certain wistfulness, she added, "I want her to see me as a good person. I want her to like most of me."

Implicit in Ruth's confession was the notion that a girl's sexual self is not admirable. And yet she knew this self was alive, curious, and even desirous. If girls acknowledge that they have feelings of desire, are they bad? If girls who think of themselves as "good" act on these "bad" feelings, must they redefine themselves as deceitful or despicable?[10] When an adolescent like Ruth begins to recognize that she has the capacity for behavior the culture labels unacceptable, how is she to judge herself? If her mother, whom Ruth hoped would see her "as a good person," could not be allowed to know this part of her, who could? She valued her relationship with Phyllis: "I think it makes me more sure of myself to know that she's behind me so no matter what I'm doing she would stand by me." Yet having said that, Ruth admitted she didn't think she could now talk comfortably about personal issues with anyone older than college age. It was to her peers that she increasingly turned for information, explanation, and advice.

Now, when sexual topics came up at home, "like maybe something happens on TV or there's a class discussion and I mention it," Ruth explained, she "sort of" talked with her parents, but withheld her true thoughts. Phyllis, accustomed to Ruth's questions, was confused by this aloofness. Ironically, just when Ruth most needed her mother to keep talking and reassuring her that it was okay to think about sex, Phyllis, not wanting to be intrusive, pulled away.

This response, in turn, reinforced Ruth's sense that it was risky to confide in her mother. If she were to ask about contraception or sexual desire, Ruth imagined that her mother would assume she was on the verge of becoming sexually active. "Maybe she knows that I have different ideas in my head when she's saying something, but I think there are other things she just has no idea about, because I don't let on knowing." Rather than endanger her relationship with her mother, Ruth chose to guard her privacy.

\*   \*   \*

Alma and Angela Parks were engaged in the same kind of distancing dance. Angela, at fifteen the rambunctious go-getter at Jefferson High, had earlier posed questions to her mom without hesitation. Now, however, she was cutting back on her inquiries "in order not to worry her." Alma Parks, however, was not backing off: "I keep talking and telling it like it is. I think if I keep doing that, they'll be going their own way but using these things they hear and remembering what I told them." Angela admitted to me that she appreciated her mom's straight talk and knew it was her way of showing she cared. But it wasn't always easy.

Alma recalled how coming to understand her adolescent daughter had been more than she bargained for. "It took me a while. . . . I still had problems. . . . Why does she function like this? Who is she? Where is she coming from? But I learned." As another mother said, "I spend more time thinking about how to deal with her now than I did the terrible twos or any of those other supposedly hard stages. I'm far more careful. . . . If I push too hard, she just clams up. Some of those little tricks seem to work better, you know, just sort of repeat back what she said."

For girls like Ruth and Angela who have passed through puberty and become aware of their own sexuality, it is not unusual to retreat quietly from heart-to-heart chats with their mothers. If communication dries up, it is not necessarily a sign that mothers are doing something wrong. As psychologist Terri Apter explains, "As a very young adult, a woman often has, towards her mother, a cooling off or brushing off phase. . . . She is a woman, too, now and an equal of her mother."[11] If there is communication, it may be only as argument. "I've learned by trial and error," said one mother. "You're never quite sure if what you say will trigger an outburst. . . . Both of us have [had to] learn to deal with this." ·

The acting out of adolescent girls may be a healthy coping strategy for them, but it is a challenge for their mothers.[12] Fifteen-year-old Tiffany Henderson, whose parents had been divorced and then reconciled, was working her way through a more volatile relationship with her mother, Marian. With her father back in the house, Tiffany worried that her mother would pull away from her. Eventually Marian wooed Tiffany back "until she understood that I wanted nothing less in our relationship than what we had when we were a single-parent family."

Through the family's upheavals, Tiffany had remained well behaved. Then, just before she turned thirteen, her life changed abruptly. It started innocently enough with a request to go to a dance. Marian said no. Her mom's excuse, Tiffany said, was that she hadn't allowed enough time to buy a dress. "So, I just decided to tell her I was going to a friend's house, and I went to the dance from there." When Marian discovered her daughter's deceit, she grounded Tiffany. Two little lies — one from the mother and one from the daughter — and thereafter Tiffany continued to act in ways guaranteed to irritate and frustrate her parents. She wasn't supposed to wear lipstick, but she would put it on at school and forget to wipe it off before Marian picked her up. She insisted on wearing "too-short" skirts to school. "I wanted to argue against everything," Tiffany recalled. "Whatever my mom said, I wanted to know WHY? I was grounded just about every week for something."

Marian was trying to provide the kind of protection and guidance she believed Tiffany needed, and increasingly Tiffany viewed it as an intrusion. While the fights were seemingly over lipstick, curfews, boys, and skirt length, they were really over power and control. Tiffany was experimenting with her new body, her new womanly self, and Marian, remembering her own adolescent missteps, was determined to keep her daughter safe. Tiffany, however, was just as determined to be independent and make her own decisions.

Tiffany's need for Marian to let go a little and Marian's counterneed to insist on protecting her daughter built up a barrier in their general communication, which spilled into conversation around sexual issues as well. Tiffany, like Ruth, was convinced that if she asked about sexual matters her mom would think that she was "nearing sex." "No matter how much I tell her," Tiffany explained, "she doesn't believe that I have the strength to determine what's going to happen for myself and no one can push me into it."

Tiffany maintained an impassive and sometimes even resistant front with her mother, but to me she conceded her mom's influence: "It's always back there, everything she's said to me." It was a common refrain: older girls wanted their mothers to trust them and to realize that conversation about sex was not going to prompt them to it. Tiffany confided that she actually agreed with almost everything her mom was saying about sex, but she didn't dare tell her that. Her silence was her small revenge for feeling as though her own voice went unheard. "I understand her perspective," she said. "But I don't think she understands mine."

Mothers' not understanding was a common theme expressed by the girls. Gerry and Carolyn Valentia eventually discovered that they needed to have a cooling-off period when tempers flared. "If cross-fire begins, one of us leaves the room. And I have learned not to feed into her," explained Gerry. "My husband says that I let her get away with too much, but I realize that she's not rational at the time. She's angry, she's upset. If she leaves the room and calms down, I calm down too, and a few seconds later, she'll come down and say, 'Well, mom . . .' and we may resume the discussion or we may not. I will usually leave it up to her."

Effective dialogue around sex during midadolescence may especially require new strategies. With girls' interests turning more to boys and "doing it," mothers such as Gerry can become very astute at determining the best times for conversation with their daughters. Gerry had learned with her older children that she had to set aside her own timetable and wait until her teen was "in the moment." She practiced the art of becoming invisible, standing at the kitchen sink putting dishes away or making dinner as Carolyn and her friends strolled in for after-school snacks and talked around the kitchen table. She rarely intruded on the girls' conversation, but she could barely keep silent the day she heard one of the girls talk about a friend "who had gone to fourth base on Friday night" — meaning she had had sex. Gerry found herself gripping the kitchen counter. "I was just so totally shocked because this girl had been in my house many times and was good friends with my children. I kept thinking, Oh no, not seventh and eighth grade. I mean are they all doing it?" Later Gerry talked to her daughter alone about what she had heard. " 'You had better be ready to deal with the consequences — physically and emotionally — if you do this,' I told her. 'It's not easy.' " After much trial and error, Gerry's strategies, such as pulling back when Carolyn became angry, being ready to listen when her daughters wanted to talk, and sometimes saying exactly what she thought, were succeeding.

Like Gerry Valentia, Samantha Brown's mother, Estelle, turned to peers' examples as a means of talking with Sam about sex. At seventeen, Sam rarely discussed sex with her mother, but she appreciated her mother's overtures when her parents found out her best friend had become pregnant. "My mother was like, 'Are you sexually active like her? If you are just tell me now and we can do whatever needs to be done.' " Sam continued, "I always thought it would be so awkward to talk to her about it, but, um, she told me that she wasn't doing it because she wanted to pry into my life but because she really cared and she didn't want me to get hurt in the long run. And I think that made a big difference because it didn't make it seem like she didn't trust me. It just seemed like she wanted to help me more."

When our girls see this distinction between caring and prying, we have succeeded at communication. What happens, though, when a teenage daughter rejects her mother's advice and becomes sexually active, as fifteen-year-old Melinda Early had done? Melinda, the tall, outspoken young woman from Jefferson, had enjoyed an easy and open relationship with her mother leading up to her teens. She had also talked intimately with her grandmother and aunts about sex. When she was thirteen, however, her mother remarried and soon Melinda had a new baby brother to take care of. Around the same time, Melinda reached puberty and began maturing rapidly. Both mom and daughter found communication harder, but Diane was convinced that she was being open and communicative: "I tell her —

I know how you get sometimes, you're a teenager and you see a boy out there. It may be the one you *like* is not the one that *should be* for you."

When I spoke with Melinda, however, I thought I was hearing about another relationship. Melinda reported that she and her mother "talked around the issues" whenever a sexual topic was introduced and that her mother "would just be like, 'Don't do that until . . .' She won't get into details." Melinda had grown more and more uneasy with these conversations. "If I asked [about sex], she would have a fit and say, 'Why do you need to know that?' She thinks if I know too much, I may want to experience it."

During Melinda's first year of high school, she began to date one young man steadily. After eighteen months, they made the decision to have sexual intercourse. Melinda was proud of the fact that she and her boyfriend first established that they cared about each other and took a long time getting to know each other. "If you do it when you barely know the person, it's just like they get what they want and then they're gone. It's not going to be like that for me, though, because it took forever. It was just the time. You can tell when it is the right time." Like many girls, Melinda had not approached her mother for guidance when the time came.

Melinda suspected Diane would be angry if she knew of her sexual activity: "If my mother knew, she would be so mad that they would probably have to rebuild the house." She admitted, echoing Ruth's words, "and she would be disappointed." As this fifteen-year-old said, "There are things that you just don't tell your mother because it's personal. She doesn't tell me about her relationships, and I wouldn't want to tell her about mine. It's something that you should keep to yourself."

She worried, however, that her grandmother, with whom she was particularly close, would find out. "She would know in a second what I am doing. She can look at you and tell you that you did something — I mean she is just that good." She continued to talk with her aunt, who frequently reminded her of the importance of female contraception and condoms. "You know how parents are overprotective about their daughters. . . . [My mother] doesn't feel comfortable telling me what she wants me to know. We talk about it, but we don't get down into it like my aunt would." Despite her secretiveness, Melinda believed that her mother suspected she was sexually active.

## Becoming Responsible for Herself

For many mothers, learning that an adolescent daughter is sexually active is the realization of their worst fear. We try to do everything to guard our girls against emotional and physical harm in adolescence. Diane Early might well have been distressed by Melinda's decision, but she would have had reason to be proud of Melinda's responsible approach to sex. Before having intercourse, Melinda visited her doctor, a woman whom she already knew, and asked for contraceptive jelly to use with her boyfriend's condoms. She talked with her friends, but she also relied on the advice of her doctor and her aunt. She was aware of the risks of pregnancy, AIDS, and other STDs. Though young in years, Melinda possessed a certain maturity. She acknowledged that having sex meant you were "growing up, getting older and have to assume more responsibility. You can't mess up if you are going to be sexually active."

And, in fact, two of the three girls in the group who were sexually active had reached their decisions with careful consideration, as their mothers had advised. Even if we can't ensure that our girls will come to us when they're deciding to engage in sex, our words and cautions do appear to have some influence on how they go about making that decision. These girls, for instance, placed a high priority on getting to know their partner well, making sure they were in a caring relationship, and using protection. As one reported with disdain, "You see a lot of relationships are kissing, kissing in the first week . . . and they end up having intercourse before they even know each other. And I was like, I'm not having that. And then after the sex and stuff, the boy tends to slip away and that's the end of the relationship. It ends before it begins."

"Some mothers feel comfortable answering questions that their daughters ask, but others feel insecure and shy about telling their child about sex, so you have to take things slowly and let them progress, or if they don't then the daughter will have to go to someone else," Melinda concluded. She trusted that Diane would someday understand her daughter's choice to become sexually active. Sounding like a mother herself, Melinda said, "For now, we'll take it one day at a time. Things will get better."

The passage through adolescence stretches both mothers and daughters. "This is like improvisational theater, only the curtain doesn't ever come down," one mother mused. Mothers with eager-to-please little girls curled up next to them holding hands suddenly find their children replaced by strange, mute creatures who glower one minute and then sit at the kitchen table insisting their mothers talk into the night. One daughter may say very little about her unfolding sexuality, while another will tell far more than her mother wants to hear. One will toss questions on the table like the morning newspaper, another will ask nothing.

But every daughter with whom I spoke was grateful when her mother reached out and let her know she was loved, supported, and understood, whether or not she expressed it to her mom. Every girl appreciated her mother's efforts to show care and concern, and, if her mother was unable to talk about sex, expressed regret. If not all daughters were willing to reveal what was on their minds, they all placed a high value on one day being able to speak openly and honestly with their moms. Each girl I met was reaching toward knowing enough, factually, socially, and emotionally, to feel responsible for herself in a relationship.

Most mothers would agree, I think, that our main objective is to raise daughters who can be independent, self-sufficient, and self-possessed. As our girls pass through adolescence, we watch as the bonds that tie us stretch further, further, further — and pray they'll never snap. How far to stretch, when to stretch, when to pull a girl close again and when to push her a little bit away is art, not science.

The events of a daughter's life at home, at school, in the world around her, and the rate of her own developmental clock determine our own dialogue and actions. Of course, we will make mistakes. But as these mothers and daughters reveal, if we love hard, talk from both the head and the heart, admit our worst mistakes, and forgive both ours and hers, the odds — even if they aren't the end result we may hope for — favor our girls' being safe. We'll never stop wanting to offer advice and encouragement, but we can take solace in thinking that eventually, with or without us, our daughters will make good decisions and live satisfying lives.

# FOUR

# Nuts and Bolts and More

## WHAT ADOLESCENT GIRLS
## KNOW ABOUT SEX

❖

**M**ary Robbins, the elegant lawyer whose vivacious daughter had schemed with me about the computer game, was getting ready to attend a parent meeting at Nottingham School titled "How to Talk to Your Child about Sex" when Vicki walked into her bedroom and told her, "You know, you don't need to go to that meeting because I know everything already." Mary went anyway, although she said her thirteen-year-old daughter "does think that she knows absolutely everything. And she certainly knows a lot more than I knew when I was twenty."

Asked "What do you think your daughter knows about sex?" the collective answer of all the mothers was "Almost everything." "There isn't anything she doesn't know," Emily Shattuck said of fifteen-year-old Katrina. "I don't see how she could not know. The TV shows and movies she sees are very explicit. . . . I'm sure she talks to her friends a great deal, and since I was a single mother and dating after my divorce and her father lives with a woman, she's been exposed to a lot." Daughters, asked to assess their own knowledge, responded in a similar fashion. Mothers were so confident their daughters understood "most all there was to know about sex," at least in theory, and daughters were so sure about the scope of their sexual knowledge, that at first it seemed our society must be doing a terrific job of sex education. When Carmen, a freshman at Jefferson, declared, "I know how to do it. . . . I know how to have sex . . . and I know the risks — AIDS, pregnancy, sexually transmitted diseases — all that. . . . I think I understand everything," I began to assume, like the mothers I interviewed, that these teenage girls did, in fact, have an amazing grasp of sex-related information. A little probing, however, revealed that their knowledge was like a puzzle sold at a yard sale for a quarter. The box looks full, but when it's time to put the pieces together, there are some glaring holes.

Whether the girls were fifteen, like Ruth, or thirteen, like Vicki, all were familiar with much of the terminology of sex and sexuality — intercourse, menstruation, masturbation, penetration, castration, oral sex, anal sex, homosexual sex, abstinence, contraception, abortion. They had amassed enough information about these terms to put on a knowing exterior, and they cared enough about teen coolness to be reluctant to admit what they weren't familiar with. I quickly learned, though, that not asking didn't always stem from a desire to appear cool. As fourteen-year-old Ingrid Shepherd explained, "I think I know pretty much everything that it occurs to me to think that I need to know — meaning, *I don't know what I don't know.*" She understood that girls don't always realize what information they're missing. For example, one of Katrina's friends, during her middle-school years, said she was relieved that her parents "had only done it three times," as evidenced by their three children, and not six times like her friend's parents who had six offspring.

This may seem laughable, but fundamental misconceptions like these are not unusual among adolescents. Girls who incorrectly believe they are well informed are unlikely to look for ways to correct misinformation. And, no matter how much factual information they possess, until they develop the ability to think abstractly and their judgment becomes mature, they can't possibly be fully aware of all that sex involves. If, in addition, we fail to emphasize at every step of girls' development that sexuality must always be addressed in the context of relationships, it becomes easy for adolescents to think that understanding the vocabulary — or even the mechanism — is the same as understanding sex.

In high school, as girls' abstract thinking skills become more developed, they generally have a better understanding of how to apply factual information to their own decisions and behaviors. If they are already sexually active, we may assume, often incorrectly, that they understand even more. Approaching sixteen, Melinda Early had been having intercourse with her long-term boyfriend, but she did not know what a clitoris was, had never heard of orgasm, and was only vaguely familiar with the term "masturbation," although she was quick to assure me "I don't do it." Girls who spend hours in front of the mirror scrutinizing their appearances often have no idea what their genitals look like. Many girls believe it is more acceptable to be touched by a young man than to touch themselves.

When, where, and how each girl learns about sex, sexuality, and her own sexual health depends, of course, on the circumstances of her life. Her own developmental patterns, the adults and organizations with which she comes into contact, the climate of her school and peer group, the media, and the culture of her community all influence what she knows and when she knows it. The girls and their mothers shared with me what they thought girls knew about the following topics: 1) human anatomy and reproduction, 2) puberty and menstruation, 3) physical risks of sexual activity, 4) contraception, 5) abortion, 6) sexual pleasures, 7) sexual orientation, and 8) emotional aspects. Their words, as well as other studies, help to broaden our understanding of precisely what adolescent girls understand about sex and sexuality.

## The Basics

### *What Girls Know about Anatomy and Reproduction*

Marian Henderson remembered when Tiffany was eight and wanted to know "the real truth about sex": "I told her that men and women have intimate relationships with one another and part of that relationship entails sex, and I described, in modest detail, what this and that are and how a woman becomes pregnant. . . . I ended with a little dose of 'But this only happens when you really love someone or you have been married to someone.'" At that point Tiffany put her hands over her ears and said, "That's enough, that's enough."

Marian's anecdote resembled those of other moms who had put away old reproduction myths about storks' dropping babies under bushes or parents' rubbing tummies, which some of them had heard when they were coming of age. As one mother noted, her daughter wouldn't have believed the cabbage-patch story for a second if she had tried it. Most of their daughters, by the time they approached puberty, knew about the nuts and bolts of anatomy and reproduction, often thanks to maternal explanations. When Ruth Rosenbloom was in fourth grade, she had insisted that her mother tell her how women have babies. Ruth's mother gave her the details, and Ruth looked at her and said, "That is the grossest thing I ever heard in my life." Phyllis was sure she had done an awful job, but she softened the blow by saying, "Well, I know it sounds gross to you, but someday it will be wonderful and beautiful — when you're married!"

Girls who are not specifically taught correct anatomical terms and functions often come away with half-truths. When 160 girls, ages thirteen to eighteen, were surveyed about their knowledge of anatomical or functional terms, they revealed major gaps in information as well as a great deal of misinformation. The only two terms that everyone knew were "anus" and "penis." They were most likely to label and correctly define the vagina, testicles, and penis, and in general they found it easier to recognize nontechnical slang terms than medically correct terminology. Less than half of the participants could correctly identify other body parts and functions, including the cervix, clitoris, and urethra. Also on the perimeters of their knowledge were such phrases as "confidential," "sexually active," and "sexually transmitted disease."[1]

Before conducting this survey, the researchers had hypothesized that adolescents who were older, were sexually active, and/or had received formal sex education would be better informed. What the study revealed, however, was that basic knowledge of reproduction and health issues was independent of these variables. Adults cannot assume that adolescents fully understand what we're talking about; we need to ask questions about their knowledge and explain our answers in words that adolescents understand — and sometimes that's not the technical language we're accustomed to.

In another survey of ninety adolescent boys and girls between the ages of thirteen and fifteen (more than half were girls), the gaps in knowledge about sexual terms were further laid bare. These teens were asked to define, in their own words, ejaculation, hormones, menstruation, ovulation, puberty, semen, and wet dreams. In an interesting twist, seventy-three mothers were also asked to participate, and the results were this: mothers and adolescent girls were most likely to define correctly menstruation and semen and least likely to define correctly ovulation and wet dreams; 88 percent of the mothers and 67 percent of the adolescent girls correctly defined menstruation. Mothers had the highest percentage of correct responses for all terms except puberty, which a higher percentage of girls defined correctly. Adolescent males had the highest percentage of incorrect definitions for all terms except wet dreams.

But what the study conveyed overall was that both boys and girls were unable to define adequately most of the seven sexual-development terms. How can we, then, expect our teens to be "prepared to engage in meaningful dialogue with peers about basic processes related to sexual behavior"?[2]

Given that most of the mothers in my project reported little or no sexual education growing up and seldom discussed sex with other women, it is likely that many women today are still not completely comfortable with anatomical definitions and the technical aspects of reproduction beyond the basics. This conclusion is bolstered by the survey that included mothers. When sex education at school is hurried or discouraged and when other informed adults fail to talk with teens about sexual matters, it is easy for girls to assume that they understand it all, when, in fact, their knowledge is patchy.

Though most early (ages ten to thirteen) and midadolescent (thirteen to sixteen) girls today generally understand the mechanics of reproduction and comprehend the way in which adults couple, the finer points seem to get lost. So much misinformation floats along the teenage grapevine that even seemingly sophisticated girls can reach improbable conclusions. Some girls in my group counseling sessions, for instance, boldly explained to me that if their periods were not yet regular, they didn't have to worry about getting pregnant. Other teens have said that they could reduce their chances of conception by not getting up quickly after sex. Adolescents consistently miscalculate the odds of conceiving without contraception. One young woman shared her belief that a girl couldn't get pregnant the first time she had sex. She might have been stunned to learn that a sexually active teenager who isn't using contraception has a 90 percent chance of becoming pregnant within a year. Another girl, oblivious to the insult of a boy's words, believed him when he told her that she couldn't get pregnant because he had already had sex once that day and had "used up all the juice." Several girls in the focus groups talked about hypothetical "safe days" but weren't sure exactly which days might be safe. To protect our girls, we must provide many sources of information so they can hear the facts presented in different ways by different people.[3]

### *What Girls Know about Puberty and Menstruation*

Technically, puberty is the stage during which a girl becomes physically capable of having a baby, launched by menarche, which traditionally occurs in early adolescence. Many mothers and daughters, however, adopt a more general definition of puberty that encompasses both the physical and the emotional changes.[4] Girls may begin to display curvy bodies — and pointed tongues — many months or even a year or two before they actually begin menstruation, and their mothers certainly consider them pubescent.

To girls, puberty is more than a rite of passage to womanhood. As one twelve-year-old explained, "You're used to your old self and then you have to adjust to your new self . . . like when your chest starts to grow." As we saw earlier, sometimes the changes, whether physical or emotional that occur in early adolescence can be quite dramatic. "Puberty? Oh, yes," one mother groaned. "My daughter became an adolescent at 8:30 P.M. on July 17, 1988." Betty Graham, a mother who had relished shopping trips with her young daughter, felt as if she had been hit between the eyes when Camille entered puberty. In her words, "puberty occurred overnight. One night when she was just thirteen, she went to one of the junior high dances. The next day she was a totally different daughter. Puberty made her a little nutsy. Until then," said Betty, "Camille and her friends had not shown much interest in boys. After the dance, boys were a prime interest. The phone started ringing and it didn't stop — it just went from call waiting to call waiting. She never even hung up. . . . She suddenly became her own person."

Betty was well informed about the importance of talking with her daughter about sexuality, but she recounted how this new person was increasingly difficult to deal with on all fronts. For the first time she saw her daughter's temper in action. "It comes on like a firestorm and then she just blows herself cool." Camille's sudden temper and sassy backtalk were making life unpleasant in the Graham household. "She says some pretty hard things, and I resent it," Betty said, but she was struggling to step back and keep a perspective on her daughter's emerging new self.

Vicki Robbins, who was just beginning puberty at thirteen, was curious about boys and watchful of how her mother and other women in her family behaved. Ingrid, who had already developed shapely breasts and hips, was delighted by her fourteen-year-old body. She had even persuaded her mom to buy her a two-piece bathing suit, which she showed off at the swimming pool. But puberty may cause some girls to cover up their new shapes. The girls in my counseling groups, for instance, preferred baggy clothes cut like cereal boxes to disguise their emerging curves. They appeared uncomfortable with the attention that their womanly bodies elicited and were doing all they could to hide the transformation.

Although we associate puberty with early adolescence, more and more girls today are showing the physical signs of puberty — pubic and body hair, breast development, the broadening of the genitalia, as well as menses — at younger ages. This is a change that girls and moms, and even some health professionals, may not be aware of or prepared for. In fact, a pediatrician in North Carolina noticed that in her practice girls in grades one to five were already showing pubic hair and breast development. In her words, "It seemed like there were too many, too young."[5] She and her colleagues and the American Academy of Pediatrics mobilized 225 clinicians in pediatric practices across the country to look further into the matter of early puberty.

In a wide-ranging study, the clinicians reported back on 17,077 girls, ages three to twelve, 90 percent of whom were white and 10 percent African-American. They discovered that by the age of eight, 48 percent of the African-American girls and 15 percent of the white girls already had some breast development, pubic hair, or both. By age seven, 27 percent of African-American girls had some secondary sexual characteristics, and just under 8 percent of white girls had evidence of breast and/or pubic hair development. The results "strongly suggest(ed) that earlier puberty is a real phenomenon and this has important clinical, education and social implications." They also noted that "more appropriate standards, taking into account racial differences, may need to be developed to define precocious and delayed puberty."[6]

These earlier physical changes make the distinction between physical and emotional puberty all the more critical.[7] Girls today are maturing at such an early age — many have sex before the age at which our grandmothers began menstruating. When girls begin puberty at seven or eight, they may look physically mature and even be emotionally charged in ways associated with adolescence, but their emotional outlook and mental development are, appropriately, those of schoolgirls.

While the softening body shifts of puberty can begin well ahead of menstruation, menarche is the moment that inevitably captures the attention of both mother and daughter. Most of the mothers recalled being frightened when they began to menstruate and were determined to guard their daughters against similar experiences. Gerry Valentia, for example, still vividly remembered how she thought she was dying when she first discovered her menstrual blood. "My mother didn't explain anything. I felt so bad about myself. . . . For my mother, menstruation was 'the curse,' and I knew I was never going to describe it that way because I think if you do, it becomes that." Gerry educated her two daughters, Carolyn and Jen, about when and how menstruation begins before the event. She showed them sanitary napkins and tampons and talked with them about the importance of bathing regularly and changing pads or tampons. She also made sure they saw menstruation as a part of normal development, not as an ailment, and assured them they could continue all their regular activities during their periods.

Once the girls began menstruating, she helped them and their father and brothers be sensitive to the accompanying changes in moods and behavior. "They don't have to tell me they're about to get their periods. The mood swings start a few days before their periods. When I see their clothes all over the floor, I think, it must be bloat, and I back off." Gerry was especially alert to her girls' hormonal surges because she remembered feeling confused and disoriented when she was growing up. "No one told me, Okay, that's a time when your face may break out or you may not feel so good about yourself. . . . I tell the girls this is just part of life. . . . Sometimes you get a little bloated or feel yucky, but you'll get over it." At the same time, she cut her daughters some slack when she thought they needed it and urged her husband to do the same. "Fathers may be harder on daughters than mothers because they don't really understand the emotional and hormonal ups and downs of female adolescent girls. I'll say 'Hon, lay off, she got her period. . . . You don't understand, but I do.'"

The conversation around menarche was probably most difficult for Rebecca Tate, who grew up in the Dominican Republic with a conservative grandmother and remembered being terrified the day she got her period. She didn't want her daughters to endure what she had experienced, yet despite her good intentions, she could not bring herself to talk with her girls. "When they were in elementary school and they asked me questions about pads and things, I just couldn't tell them the truth. I joked about it or told them stories," she said.

When her daughter Cecile began to develop breasts and pubic hair at eleven, however, Rebecca realized she could no longer postpone discussing menstruation. "I knew what to tell her but I just found it so emotionally upsetting." She forged ahead nonetheless, explaining to Cecile, "You wanted to know what these things [pads and tampons] were for all this time, and I didn't tell you. I'd make a joke. But now I want to tell you what they are for because any day now — probably between now and when you are twelve — you will be having a period and you will see blood on your pants. All you have to do is come to me," she said. "If you're not at home, go to the nurse at school and tell her."

Ingrid Shepherd was so well informed and prepared for womanhood that when she discovered, at age eleven, the start of menstruation while away at summer camp, she took out the supplies her mother had packed and continued on with her camp activities. "My mom had told me all about it and she had given me pads and stuff," Ingrid recounted. "[At camp] I woke up one morning, and I'm like, 'Oh, cool!' I went to my trunk and I got my stuff out. I mean they expected me to go to the nurse or something." When her mom came, "I told her and she was like, 'Oooh.' . . . And I mean, like within about twenty minutes, it's like everybody my mom knew knew. . . . She asked me before if she could tell. She just wanted to make sure."

Thirteen-year-old Jenny King was also glad to have joined the ranks of the girls "in the know" at age twelve, but she was notably less enthusiastic and saw menstruation as unfair for women. "I didn't like it and I still don't. . . . I guess it's a good thing, but it's a pain in the butt," she complained. "I don't [have] cramps or anything. It's just . . . my friends and I, we talk about how unfair it is. That we get, you know, the period and the guys get — they basically get nothing. . . . And it's like the girls have to worry about this." To her mind, boys were lucky: "Their voices get deeper, they get taller, their *thing* gets bigger, but girls, you have to worry about pads, tampons, douches, whatever. . . . Girls have it harder than guys," she concluded.

Even when mothers have done their best to prepare their daughters for menstruation, girls may have unexpected reactions when they see menstrual blood for the first time. Phyllis Rosenbloom, one of the most forthcoming mothers on sexual topics, thought she had vigilantly prepared Ruth for menstruation. One night, though, Ruth watched a television movie about a man who urinated blood and ended up dying of cancer. The next morning Ruth came into her parents' bedroom, hysterical and crying, "There's something wrong, there's something wrong."

"Finally," Phyllis explained, "I got it out of her what was happening. She woke up with blood on her pajamas and was sure she was dying of cancer. It took me a while to convince her she had just begun her period."

Menstruation is not the same for all girls. Some will experience occasional cramps, which can be eased by exercise, a heating pad, or over-the-counter muscle relaxants. Many, like Ingrid and Jenny, experience little or no discomfort and continue easily with their day's activities. It is not uncommon for girls to worry about how much blood they are losing or about the color of the blood. They may be surprised, for instance, by the brownish, clotty character of menstrual fluid or shocked by what appears to be a great amount of blood loss. In general, though, an average period produces about one to three ounces of blood, the equivalent of two to four tablespoons, in a mixture of blood, tissue, and mucus, which can be absorbed by six to eight pads or tampons per day. Girls of any age can use tampons, but because it may take some effort to learn how to insert them correctly, some moms caution against them. Also, some girls just prefer pads when they first begin to menstruate.[8]

Beyond the basics, less well known is that during the first year or so, irregular menstrual cycles are quite common and not a cause for worry. An irregular period does not mean, however, that a girl who becomes sexually active can ignore contraception. Also, girls who participate in high-endurance sports may lose body fat to the point that their periods become irregular.

Girls may not realize that the way they view menstruation may influence how it affects them physically. Certainly some young women experience very real menstrual discomfort because of chemical changes in the uterus, and noting the effect of psychological influences isn't meant to belittle that tangible pain. But a Wellesley College study that included 600 middle- to upper-middle-class girls in grades six through nine disclosed that "adequate preparation for menstruation affects girls' attitudes, contributes to positive feelings about their menstruation and is associated with the reporting of fewer symptoms of menstrual distress." This positive attitude, the same survey observed, is not helped by product information "that emphasizes menstruation as a hygienic crisis and urges girls to try to 'act normal' so that no one will know, thus implying that having a period is somewhat abnormal or includes the risk of acting abnormally."[9]

One final note: the 1996 Boston Marathon, in which front-runner Uta Pippig approached the finish line with blood trickling down her leg, offers a poignant example of the ambivalence many in this country still feel about young women acting "normally" during menstruation and the images girls have to confront. Pippig's decision to keep running in spite of the blood provoked a range of comments. Some spoke of how brave and wonderful she was to continue; others found it shocking and distasteful to see a woman so publicly ignore her menstrual blood and thought she should have dropped out. For many women, Pippig's crossing the finish line showed that menstruation is no deterrent either to effort or success.[10]

## Beyond the Basics

### *What Girls Know about*
### *the Physical Risks of Sexual Activity*

When Camille Graham changed overnight from a "sweet little girl to pain in the neck," her mother started to worry about more than a constantly busy phone. Concerns about their daughters' becoming sexually active were commonly expressed by the mothers I spoke with. Betty Graham thought it inevitable that Camille would now feel pressure from her friends to become sexually active. To counter peer influence, Betty tried to discern what exactly her daughter knew and what she needed to know. She found out a lot by paying close attention to Camille's jokes and the conversations between Camille and her friends when she drove them to school. "One recent joke Camille told me was really gross and dirty, with all kinds of swear words and expressions," she recalled. "There is a great temptation to tell her this kind of language is inappropriate, but you have to resist. . . . I think these jokes and the conversation in the car is her way of signaling to me: 'Look what I know.' "

Most of the girls understood that if they had sexual intercourse, especially without using contraceptives, they were placing themselves at risk for getting pregnant and for contracting AIDS. For some, friends' experiences provided pointed lessons. When Samantha was sixteen, for instance, one of her best friends became pregnant. Samantha watched her friend's difficulties with growing awareness and concern. "I think about how responsible you have to be. You have to be really positive that having sex is what you want to do, and if it is, then you have to take actions to keep yourself from getting hurt by being sexually active, like using condoms and some other birth control. If you get pregnant, you would have to make sure you have some way to support yourself." Samantha seemed to weigh her friend's dilemma when she added, "I just know that I'm not ready to be that serious or have those kinds of responsibilities."

In general, my interviews and other research reveal that teens, although aware of the general dangers of sex, don't appreciate their *own* vulnerability. Despite the fact that nearly one million young women under twenty become pregnant each year, and 80 percent of those pregnancies are unplanned, none of the girls I spoke with could imagine themselves as one of that group.[11] "I just didn't think I would get pregnant" are words spoken by countless teen moms or pregnant girls. One of the pregnant teens in a focus group told other participants that she used to see friends walking down the street with strollers, and she'd say to herself, "That's not going to be me." The young woman put her hand on her stomach. "Now look at me. . . . Guess I shouldn't have spoken so soon."

Pregnancy is no longer the only major concern. "It used to be 'Don't get pregnant,' " Phyllis Rosenbloom observed, "but now we're discussing AIDS. It's a life or death situation." Cybil Mason advised Bettina, "Before you ever have sex with anyone, you march them down and have an AIDS test. I told her that's what I am going to do. . . . It's just not worth it. It's a one-act death."

Everyone, daughters and moms, understood that the stakes were high when it came to AIDS. The disease no longer seemed like a distant scourge that plagued only strangers; most families had a friend, acquaintance, or even a relative with a connection to AIDS. The death of a dear family friend of the Rosenblooms from the disease had prompted many family discussions, and Phyllis felt this had helped her daughters become better informed. No mother wanted to take the chance of failing to impress on her daughter the importance of this danger, and every daughter understood that having sex meant using a condom.

Yet girls tended to pull away from the subject. "I know, I know, I know," one girl protested to her mother. "I have heard this stuff a thousand times and I am not going to get AIDS." Some thought the risk was overstated. Katrina's mom, Emily Shattuck, expressed consternation about all the talk of AIDS. "Even in elementary school they sent a pamphlet home from school that dealt with AIDS, and they expected us to sit down and talk with our school-age kids about anal sex and homosexuality. That was really upsetting. . . . I just wonder what is left."

Despite her mother's concerns, fifteen-year-old Katrina welcomed the information provided by her school and others on AIDS. She thought it was a very important subject that girls needed to be aware of and that parents should explain it to their teenagers. "Parents," she said, "are just plain crazy if they're not talking about AIDS with their kids, especially if parents sense that their children don't have a clear understanding of something as frightening as AIDS."

Perhaps surprisingly, the girls were more specific than their mothers about the importance of contraception in preventing disease. For example, when fifteen-year-old Tiffany Henderson discussed the preparations necessary for her to become sexually active, she said, "I would use contraceptives. . . . I don't know if I would use a pill, but I would use something and he would have to use a condom too." Their concerns about HIV and AIDS were realistic: in 1996 alone, health officials identified 2,574 known cases of AIDS among teens ages thirteen to nineteen. However, "nearly 8 times as many young adults, ages twenty to twenty-four, were diagnosed during the same period . . . and the majority were infected during their teens."[12]

The societal emphasis on AIDS has made teenagers more aware of the danger, but it has also increased the demand for sex education curriculums that teach only abstinence. This approach fails to educate teens about all aspects of AIDS transmission and, just as important, about other STDs.[13] When asked what they knew about the harmful consequences of sexual intercourse, the girls' answers were usually a short litany: "pregnancy, AIDS, and other sexually transmitted diseases." It is easy to assume that adolescent girls who come of age hearing about AIDS also know about other sexually transmitted diseases, but this was not the case among girls I spoke with.

Sexual diseases such as gonorrhea, chlamydia, genital warts, hepatitis, herpes, and syphilis are far more prevalent among teens than AIDS is. When teenage girls were tested for STDs in a recent study, three of ten who were sexually active were infected with chlamydia, a bacterial disease that causes inflammation of the cervix, signaled by itchiness, burning, and occasional discharge. Untreated, it can lead to infertility. Gonorrhea is another STD, for which sexually active teenage women are at particular risk. In fact, 63 percent of all the gonorrhea cases in this country in 1992 were in young people ages ten to twenty-four. It is a harsh truth that three million teens become newly infected with some sexually transmitted disease each year, and these diseases can cause girls lasting damage. It is not enough to caution only against AIDS.[14]

The adolescent community at large displays a lack of knowledge of STDs. In a recent survey of 500 teenagers, for example, of those who said they had first learned about STDs in school, 42 percent could not name any sexually transmitted disease other than AIDS. Only 23 percent could identify genital herpes. And only 12 percent reported learning about STDs from a family member.[15]

One of the other sad ironies surrounding concern about AIDS is that it has led some teens to consider oral sex as a safe alternative to intercourse. Phyllis Rosenbloom, one of the frankest mothers of the group, remembered an evening when she and her daughters were chatting alone at dinner. "The girls started trying to bring up a topic with me, but neither of them could say it out loud. They didn't want to use the term 'oral sex.' Eventually, I guessed what they were asking about. Then they told me that this is what the boys wanted to do in place of intercourse — it was safer and the girls could still remain virgins." Phyllis was furious that boys were suggesting this as a safe and attractive alternative. "I told them so, told them not to buy into the idea that oral sex was safe and that it demanded a condom as well." She was shocked when both daughters told her, "But that's not what the boys want." Phyllis pried further. Did they know other girls who were having unprotected oral sex? Yes, was the swift reply. Later Phyllis heard from some of her friends who had teenage sons that the boys felt girls were pressuring *them* to have oral sex.

Such misconceptions extend beyond the Rosenblooms' kitchen table. According to a 1994 survey, 26 percent of a nationally representative sample of high school students had engaged in oral sex and 4 percent in anal sex. A fifteen-year-old girl who attended a private school in Manhattan explained, "For the people I know, sexual intercourse is a humongous thing. It's risky, and it's a big deal. But oral sex doesn't seem like sex. People may see the first time as a rite of passage, but after that, it's nothing much. A friend told me she'd done it to a boy last weekend, and I didn't even think to ask if she'd used a condom." She added, "but if she were having intercourse, I'd make her promise me that she would protect herself."[16]

According to this study, "boys, too, perceive a fundamental difference between intercourse and oral sex." One fourteen-year-old boy reported, "Everybody understands that intercourse is dangerous and that it requires a real commitment," but he added that "oral sex did not necessarily imply a real relationship." Another survey of Los Angeles high school students revealed that among those who counted themselves virgins, 10 percent had engaged in oral sex, and boys and girls were equally likely to be the receiving partner.[17]

The founder of the Adolescent AIDS Prevention Program at Mount Sinai Medical Center in New York City noted that as early as fifth and sixth grade, youngsters begin asking questions about oral sex because they have heard about it and are curious. "By seventh grade, they want to know if it's really safer sex, and what are the mechanics. For girls, 'Do you spit or do you swallow?' is a typical seventh-grade question." This health educator, who sees many generational and cultural differences in attitudes about sex, concluded that oral sex is most widely accepted among white middle-class adolescents who consider it less risky than intercourse — failing to understand that AIDS *can* be transmitted by oral sex.[18]

Teenagers like to believe they can manipulate statistics with wishful thinking. They understandably want to spread their wings and experience what the world has to offer. We would like to not deny them many of the joys of youth, but the world our teens are living in is, unfortunately, more precarious than the one we grew up in, and because the perils have multiplied, our girls' awareness must be more acute.

### What Girls Know about Contraception

The word Angela Parks chose when asked what came to mind when she thought about sexuality was "contraceptives." She explained that she'd been doing her own contraceptive research. Not yet sexually active herself at fifteen, Angela guessed she would wait "until I'm married or really care about someone and we have a commitment between us." Yet several of her friends who claimed to be using condoms had gotten pregnant, and Angela had decided "to check out the situation so I'll know the truth." The truth, she concluded, was that "you've got to go both ways. Girls should use something like a diaphragm with jelly, the sponge or foam and guys need to use a condom." Angela knew that many health care providers recommended birth control pills, but she opposed the pills because she thought they "altered the natural course of females too much."

The younger girls in the study were not especially interested in knowing the fine points of different methods of contraception. Jenny

King, at thirteen, was sure "no one my age can really love anybody enough to have sex." But fourteen-year-old Ingrid was becoming more interested in the particulars of sex. Having heard a lot about jellies and diaphragms, she turned to her mother for a more detailed explanation. "She told me what she knew and then showed me hers [diaphragm]."

According to Ingrid, her mother wasn't familiar with some of the new products available on the market, which only heightened Ingrid's resolve to get more information. "The next time we were at the store, I stopped by the contraceptives that were next to the pads. I picked up some of the stuff my mom didn't know about, and I just stood there reading. This guy kept looking at me, but I just kept reading." Later, when Ingrid was recapping for her friends at school what a diaphragm was, her science teacher walked by and asked if they were talking about the importance of taking deep breaths! Ingrid had gained a reputation among her peers as the girl who had the straight scoop on sexual stuff. If Ingrid didn't know the answers right away, everyone trusted that she would go home, corner her mom, get the real story, and tell them the next day.

Samantha at seventeen had given a great deal of thought to different types of birth control. Sam was certain she would go to her doctor for birth control and that her partner would be ready to use condoms before trying intercourse. "We would have to talk in advance about what would happen." She was adamant that if a girl could not talk easily with her partner about contraception, she was not ready to engage in sex with him.

Katrina, two years younger than Samantha, similarly stressed the importance of birth control if she decided to become sexually active and said she would plan to visit her doctor to obtain it. When she was younger, her mother had often taken Katrina along on visits to the gynecologist and had once explained that the visit was for a birth control device. "I told Katrina we wanted to limit the size of our family, that we liked it this size and that birth control let us keep it the way we liked it." Recently Katrina had visited her own gynecologist, and her mother was relieved that she had established a relationship with someone with whom she felt comfortable in discussing contraception. Katrina, like Ingrid and Angela, had also spent time at the grocery store and pharmacy inspecting the various over-the-counter products.

The majority of mothers I talked with gave their daughters a clear message: Don't be sexually active, at least while you are in high school. But if you are, be sure to protect yourself. Melinda, who was already having sex with her boyfriend, said of her mother, "She just says, 'Whenever you decide to have sex — which I know isn't going to be anytime soon — like when you are married — make sure you protect yourself.' " This was typical of maternal messages: mothers were more likely to caution daughters about taking care than to spell out specifically how that care could be taken.

In general, girls who desired specific information about the effectiveness and the advantages and disadvantages of various methods of contraception — pills, diaphragm, foams, jellies, injectable hormones like Depo-Provera, or implants — lacked easy access to this information. Nottingham School had integrated some information about contraceptives into its growth education classes, but at Jefferson, girls were learning about them from their peers or occasionally from a counselor or nurse who was willing to take a risk and talk to students if asked. The girls might have been surprised to learn that the pill is 97 percent effective when used as prescribed, condoms are 88 percent effective, and that next to sterilization, Norplant and the injectable contraceptive Depo-Provera are the most effective.[19]

Mothers who say "If you're going to be sexually active, then come to me and we'll go to the clinic for birth control" think they are being forthright. But this approach requires an adolescent daughter to lean across the kitchen table and say, "Okay, mom, now is the time." It speaks to exceptional trust and open communication when daughters can do this. Most girls, no matter how close they are to their mothers, will not come home and say, "Well, I've decided. I'm going to become sexually active, and I would like you to help me with birth control." In fact, none of the girls said they would take this approach with their moms when the time arrived.

Then there is the male point of view to consider. When a group of urban adolescent boys was asked about the likelihood that an adolescent girl would get pregnant if she had intercourse, several thought teens were less likely to get pregnant without contraception than adults, as though teens had some special membership in a pregnancy prevention program. When asked how many of them had practiced withdrawal when they had no condom or other contraception at hand, only 20 percent of the group said they had. They also reported that the first time they had sex, they were not prepared — "it just happened."[20]

Girls acknowledge that many adults believe the only safe sex is no sex. They know that many parents and religious institutions preach abstinence until marriage. But something inordinately compelling makes the majority of teens overlook these messages. They see that people like sex, talk about it, think about it, desire it, and engage in it. For many, the pleasure component of sex remains a mystery — and in the mystery lies part of the attraction. What will it feel like? Will it be as good as it seems in the movies? What does an orgasm feel like? Can girls even have orgasms?

When a young woman hears from her parents and other important adults in her life that she should abstain from sexual activity, but is convinced she is ready for it, she faces an agonizing dilemma. Either she disobeys her parents and endangers her relationship with them, or she subsumes her own desires and sense of self. Given the importance of relationships for women, a girl in this situation may feel enormous emotional upheaval. Even if she has ready access to birth control, navigating through these conflicting demands and desires can be painful.

A girl who sets out to equip herself with contraception may be forced to acknowledge that she intends to disobey her parents or her religious teachings. To obtain birth control pills (used by slightly more than half of sexually active girls), she must visit a physician (and usually incur a bill), obtain a prescription, visit a pharmacy, and pay for the pills. Pills, diaphragms, Norplant, and contraceptive hormone shots are not available over the counter. If, instead, she allows herself to be carried away in the moment with no contraception, swept up by hormones — or by alcohol — then in an odd way she may feel her behavior is not intentional and her guilt is of a lesser order.[21]

Many of the messages from moms and other adults to teens about sex indirectly reward girls who abdicate planning for their own best interests.[22] Our society sometimes seems to have a more forgiving attitude toward those who allow themselves to become victims of their hearts or hormones than those who address their sexual desires honestly and seek out contraception in advance of intimacy.

### What Girls Know about Abortion

Moms' and daughters' convictions concerning abortion ran the gamut, but everyone had definite opinions on the topic. Some of their comments were deeply personal, whereas others were guided by religious beliefs. Most focused on the decision-making process and on the right or wrong of abortion rather than on a dilemma that had entered their lives. Carmen Rankin, raised in her mother's Catholic household, expressed her firm opinion about what a pregnant girl ought to do. "I think you should wait until you're married, but if you get pregnant when you're a teenager, you should have the baby whether you give it up for adoption or not. I don't think abortion is right . . . absolutely do not believe in it even if you're raped. I think depriving a baby from life is awful. I know my sister — the first time she had sex she got pregnant and she was twenty-two — could have had an abortion. And I see the baby now, and the baby is so beautiful." Her mother used similiar words.

The Shattucks stood at the opposite end of the spectrum, reflecting the deep fissures in society at large. Emily Shattuck was sure that Katrina would go to her doctor and receive contraception if she were thinking about becoming sexually active. But if she did become pregnant, Emily said, "I know that she would have an abortion because we have talked a great deal about this." Her older daughter had acted in a high school play with a teenage mother who often brought her new baby to play practice. When the girls started gushing over how cute the baby was at a family dinner one night, Emily laid down her rules. Though their friend's parents might be supportive and help take care of the baby, her girls should not expect the same of her. She told them in no uncertain terms, "If you don't want to have an abortion, then you had better be ready to take care of the child, because I work and I'm not willing. I would encourage you to have an abortion; it's one thing to be philosophically against abortion, but it's another thing to go through with a pregnancy, keep the child, and visit the consequences on someone else."

Katrina articulated the same views as her mom about contraception, abortion, and premarital sex. "We are real big pro-choicers," she told me. "I wrote a term paper on it, and we always talk about it." Angela Parks, at fifteen, though philosophically opposed to abortion, suspected she would have one if necessary. "If I got pregnant, my mother would hit the roof. . . . She doesn't believe in abortion and I don't believe in abortion either. But I would get one the next day, even if it's a school day. I think I would cry a lot because I know I'd feel it was my fault." Again, the daughter's words paralleled her mother's views. Alma Parks had no intention of letting a mistaken pregnancy derail her daughter from her goals.

As these stories suggest, the girls I interviewed talked about abortion in terms that reflected their family's values and focused on moral and social dynamics. The specifics of when, how, and where a girl might obtain an abortion were seldom mentioned. Although twenty-two states now require parental consent for girls under eighteen to have an abortion, only a few girls were aware of what was required by their state or where abortions were performed.[23]

Most girls, although certainly not all, seemed to feel that abortion was undesirable, but that if they became pregnant in high school, they would have one. They believed it would be a very difficult decision. Ingrid Shepherd, who, like her mother, thought abortion was an acceptable choice for a pregnant unwed teen, added, "I think people should really understand that abortion is not a form of birth control — the general public needs more knowledge on this." The adolescent girls in the focus groups had very mixed feelings about abortion. Some thought they would be encouraged by their partner to have one if they were to get pregnant. On the other hand, they were very disapproving of girls who had had abortions and mainly rejected it as a reasonable option for themselves.

I encountered one noteworthy exception to this widespread ambivalence. The one Maternity Care Coalition focus group that con-
sisted of all boys expressed uniform enthusiasm. These boys were "all
for abortion" because they felt unready to be responsible for a family
and provide for a child. However, their unwillingness to become fathers did not make them want to understand more about contraception or to advocate abstinence.

What struck me time and again when discussing abortion with
moms and daughters was how different it felt from conversations
about every other subject. Unlike pregnancy, AIDS, or even rape,
abortion was a topic that most mothers and daughters were not comfortable with. Their attitude seemed to be, If we just leave this alone
and don't talk about it, maybe we won't ever have to deal with it. I began to realize that nowhere is this topic considered safe. Schools avoid
it in sex education; health care providers do very little to educate teens
about contraception and abortion, even though girls have a legal right
to such information; and parents are reluctant to discuss anything
more than their moral position.[24] This means that most of what teens
glean about abortion, they learn from their peers and the media. The
possibility that they might someday have to decide whether or not to
have an abortion was disconcerting to the girls, and they wanted very
much to avoid making such a decision — let alone figuring out the lo-
gistics of arranging for one.

### Sexual Pleasures

Angela Parks's words capture many girls' thoughts about sexual pleasure. When I asked about the gaps in her knowledge about sex, she
said, "Probably the pleasure, truthfully speaking. I don't know, I'm just
dumbfounded at that because I have never gone into that. I mean, I
can tell you many things that I've read and things my friends have told
me of their pleasure, but I really can't say it's a pleasure because I
haven't been through it." Now that Angela had grown specifically curious about the sexual experience, her mother had begun to portray sex
in more negative tones. But Angela, like most girls in midadolescence
who are bursting with hormones, wasn't buying it.

Sex was something they liked to think about, talk about with their friends, and fantasize doing. Two of the three girls who were sexually active said sex was a very nice part of their lives. They were not, each explained carefully, having sex because they felt pressured by their boyfriends but because they found it satisfying, enjoyable, and a natural expression of their relationships.

Most of the mothers said that sexual pleasure was the most difficult topic to address with their girls, but they felt it was important for their daughters to know something it. However, they worried that if they shared their own feelings about sexual pleasures, their girls would be more eager to become sexually active. Thus they believed the safest route was to focus on the risks of emotional harm from an intimate relationship as well as the potential physical dangers. Tiffany, for one, had picked up on the warning not to get sidetracked from her goals, explaining that she wasn't ready for sex because "I don't want to lose my focus."

### What Girls Know about Sexual Orientation

Our teens are becoming increasingly exposed to homosexuality through the media. But being exposed to this issue through television and movies is obviously not the same as understanding it fully when it touches friends, family, or even oneself. In my study, no girl mentioned homosexual fantasies, the dreams or exploration that heterosexual girls may normally experience and yet may find alarming or shameful. However, in two families the issue of homosexuality arose with particularly personal overtones. In one family the older daughter had claimed, when she was a teenager, to be a lesbian, and her admission had led to a family crisis. Now, at twenty-two, she had a child and planned to marry the father. In her mother's words, the girl had "outgrown her impulse."

Katrina and Emily Shattuck, who had easily joked about every sexual subject, became quite serious when the conversation turned to homosexuality. Katrina's older sister, a high school senior, was in a relationship with another woman, and this was causing heated arguments in their family. "My father thinks it's a perversion," Katrina explained. "My mother thinks it's wrong; it's not natural. My mom and my sister really get into it."

Katrina was troubled and confused by the family uproar and worried about her sister. "I try to get involved and even out the odds, but I just get my head ripped off. And I end up getting upset and leaving the room. Now I just try to distance myself from all of this." But that approach wasn't working. Katrina spoke affectionately of her sister and wanted to support her, saying, "Whatever makes you happy is okay with me." On the other hand, she confessed to her sister that she wasn't really comfortable with homosexuality and sometimes felt ashamed of her relationship. After that admission, Katrina "really felt bad because I knew that it was upsetting to her, and in a way, even though I was being honest with myself, I felt like it made her feel even more upset."

Particularly hard for Katrina was not being able to discuss her sister's relationship with her friends. "We live in such a homophobic town," she said morosely. "I tried to bring this topic up once, and my friends just didn't understand. . . . Someone's always making a rude comment, and I'll say, 'You have no right making that comment. How would you even know? Have you ever known someone who is homosexual?' I really get on the warpath about it."

Her sister's relationship had also led Katrina to question same-gender friendships. She had always taken her friendships with girls for granted, but now she wondered about the differences between friendship with a girl and a more loving relationship. Katrina had watched her sister's interaction with a young woman whom she initially assumed was just a good friend. Katrina explained, "Her friend would come over and we'd hang out, and they were really honest and close with each other. Now, as I think back, that's not the way 'just friends' behave, that's the way people act who are sexually involved." She continued, "This just blew my interpretation of friendship, and that bothers me a lot. What's most difficult is that I can't really discuss it with anyone."

The other mothers and daughters had little to say about homosexuality. It seemed that unless it touched their lives directly, moms and daughters were comfortable overlooking it in their whole dialogue about sex. One mother described her daughter as having "extreme homophobia," but she didn't think those feelings were problematic. Another girl recounted her unease during a visit with a woman minister who led the church's youth group. "I was sitting in her office talking one day, and she told me I reminded her of herself when she was my age. That's when I said, 'Whoops, gotta go.' I wouldn't want to say definitely that she was coming on to me, but she just seemed too friendly, and I didn't have good vibes, so I left." Though her intuition may have been correct, it's more likely that a certain degree of homophobia led her to misinterpret what was a caring, reaffirming gesture.

Homosexuality is a difficult and perplexing topic for parents and teens to discuss. Many recent memoirs have mentioned the denial, anger, guilt, fear, and sadness expressed by parents to daughters who attempt to discuss their lesbian feelings. Some parents insist that their daughters are in a stage they will outgrow, and in fact it is not unusual for an adolescent girl to wonder about same-sex experimentation. However, many people who have studied sexual orientation agree that when a teen says she thinks she is a lesbian and a parent responds with a comment like "Oh, it's just a phase," they risk undermining her self-esteem and dismissing a very important aspect of her self-understanding. It is crucial for parents to treat such statements with respect and caring.[25]

Teenage girls who struggle with the burden of feeling different in their sexual desires need understanding and acceptance from family and peers. If a daughter is questioning her sexual orientation, the family should work toward ensuring her psychological stability and self-esteem. Nothing hurts a child as much as anger and rejection from loved ones, and as in Katrina's case, that hurt can extend to siblings as well. When, in spite of her own ambivalence, Katrina told her sister she wanted her to feel okay being who she was, she was affirming her respect and affection for her sister. Katrina's support offers a model for us all.

### *What Girls Know about the Emotional Components of Sex*

What Ingrid felt unsure about in seventh grade was the emotional aspect of sexual relationships. Though seventh-grade sex education class "helped a lot because we had a lot of discussions about relationships," the issue remained understandably hard to get a handle on. Finally she approached her mom one day and said, "Exactly what do you mean by this psychological stuff causing harm?" As she recalled it, "My mom said, 'If you're that intimate with a person and then that person dumps you and goes on to another person, that could hurt a lot.'"

Evelyn Shepherd seized the chance to underscore for Ingrid the intangible dangers of sex: "Any time you are in a sexual relationship, that is a tremendous intimacy, a tremendous vulnerability. . . . Is that a risk you are willing to take? I'm not coming from the viewpoint of pregnancy, AIDS, STDs. I'm talking about psychologically. Psychologically there is a risk." Ingrid still couldn't fathom the kind of pain her mom described, but she concluded, "If there is this psychological effect, as I have heard many people say, I'm not ready for it. I'm just not ready to deal with that."

Tiffany, at fifteen, also believed that the emotional risks outweighed the benefits of becoming sexually involved. "I just figured," she explained, "that I would maybe care about the person and he wouldn't really care about me. Or I would just sort of like lose it all and not be able to focus because I'd be thinking about what happened and about the guy all the time. I think I'd just better wait till I'm older." Like Ingrid and Tiffany, most of the other girls trusted their mothers' advice regarding the potential for "damaging emotional consequences" of sexual activity, and for the moment most were content with the simpler pleasures of romance.

Katrina described the emotional highs that can make even first crushes so exciting when sex is not a consideration. She and a group of friends had gone to a dance, where she met a guy. When the dance turned dull, she and her friends left. "We were just walking around town, and he had his arm around me," she recalled. "I was literally swept off my feet. . . . You know, he was so nice and it was also just the night itself." She continued, "Nothing happened. I just had a really good time. The next day I thought maybe this was just my imagination — maybe I'm going crazy. Then I heard that he was still going out with another girl. I was like, Don't tell me. But I was happy that night. Even if it only lasted for a few hours, you would like to bottle that feeling."

Katrina had had just a glimpse of the thrill of romance and the letdown of disappointment. What girl, after all, can imagine the full force of rejection until she has given her heart away and found it returned with a no-thank-you note? Who can really comprehend the high stakes until faced with the consequences of a few moments of play? Tiffany was afraid to lose her focus; Ingrid was wary of unknown dangers. Katrina had a whiff of disappointment. Melinda, who dared to risk deceiving and disappointing her mother, spoke more of her mother's likely reaction than of the joys of sex. But Tiffany also knew she wanted to be hugged, Ingrid liked being admired at the pool, and Melinda felt that engaging sexually with her boyfriend was right and reasonable.

Making sure their daughters would understand the emotional components of a sexual relationship came up time and again in conversations with mothers, who generally did not think their girls were currently capable of handling the emotions. Carolyn Valentia's mom had told her, "For every action, there is a reaction. Are you ready to deal with this emotionally?" Gerry Valentia confided she would be very worried if Carolyn were having sex at fourteen: "It's a serious commitment . . . because the emotions that you will experience are so strong that it really clouds your mind."

The girls I spoke with possessed a wealth of information about menstruation, puberty, and contraception. But in midadolescence and even late adolescence the more abstract and multifaceted components of sex were still mysterious to them: all the emotions and nuances that make up a relationship, whether heterosexual or same-sex. With so much information and misinformation at our girls' fingertips, mothers and others have an invaluable role to play in filling in the gaps and helping our daughters make sense of it all.

# FIVE

# Beyond
## *Beverly Hills 90210*

### WHERE GIRLS GET
### THEIR INFORMATION

........................❖........................

**I**f there were a generic recipe for how girls today find out about sex, it might read:

> 1 mother
> Half-dozen best friends
> 1–10 cups of television pureed and added to taste
> 1 sex education class
> Assorted magazines, crumbled into bite-size pieces
> 2 cups movies
>
> *Sprinkle the above liberally with:*
> Book pages in large chunks
> 1 cup older sister or cousin
> Dash of father
> Assorted peers to flavor as needed

Different families, different recipes. Some stir in aunts and grandparents, while others skimp on the television and increase religion; some spike the recipe with boyfriends or dirty books. But most sex education, as we have seen, begins with one mother. Perhaps not surprisingly, the sexual socialization of children is considered part of a mother's duties, and sexuality is still viewed as a "woman's issue"; that is, girls need to know about menstruation, pregnancy, birth control, lactation, and menopause, all of which fall squarely in the female domain. What's more, research reveals that women are generally more comfortable and skilled than men in dealing with value-laden issues and, in addition, daughters perceive mothers to be more emotionally expressive, more affectionate, more available, and less punitive than the men in their lives.[1]

Even during adolescence, as girls begin to separate from their mothers, they retain an important connection. Those girls who pulled back from closeness during midadolescence still spoke of wanting their mothers to approve of their sexual selves: their mothers' opinions continued to matter significantly. A daughter may identify with her mother for a host of reasons, the most significant being their common fate as women, but the girls I talked to, especially younger ones, fondly mentioned a certain camaraderie — and trust — shared with their moms. If mothers are such valuable resources in the communication process, what strategies have they found useful in interactions with their daughters about sexual issues?[2]

## The Importance of Mothers

Mothers used three main approaches for getting their messages across, and their different tacks met with varying levels of success. The most valued strategy among moms, many of whom remembered their own adolescent ignorance, was direct and open communication. In fact, 75 percent believed they were communicating directly and openly with their daughters when it came to sex. They talked about trying to leave the door wide open and making sure their girls felt comfortable discussing any topic. Moreover, those moms *initiated* conversation. As Alma Parks said, "I talk for real. I don't hide [any]thing with my children." Those moms who spoke openly also tended to have begun talking about these issues early on, as soon as a girl's curiosity was piqued.

But were daughters ranking their communication with moms as high? Not quite. Only one-half of the girls, as opposed to three-quarters of mothers, thought their conversations were direct and open. Those girls who viewed their communication in a good light also noted that their moms had begun talking about sex at an early age. But why this discrepancy in moms' and daughters' descriptions? Girls, it appeared, were defining "direct and open" communication in very different ways from their moms. To the daughters' minds, "direct and open" didn't just mean an open door or even initiating conversation; it hinged on whether their moms *listened* to them. Whereas mothers who warned their daughters about the risks surrounding sexual activity saw their approach as direct and open, daughters expected much more. If they felt their moms weren't actually listening to their words and were not giving some indication that they understood what their daughters were thinking, then there were problems. In the simplest terms, it had to be two-way communication coupled with understanding before the girls would consider it an open process. Conversely, mothers were likely to judge their communication skills based on whether or not *they* could speak comfortably with their girls about sexuality rather than on their daughters' reaction or participation.

For moms and daughters who did not have open communication — and even for many who did — "talking around the issues" turned out to be an effective and sometimes more comfortable way of engaging in a conversation. This meant speaking in general terms. Rather then telling her daughter "Don't get pregnant," a mother would turn to another girl's problem as an example of what not to do. Typically daughters read between the lines, even when moms spoke in circuitous ways. As one daughter explained, "We don't get all down to the nitty-gritty 'cause I know she's not gonna go that far." But the messages registered. Talking around the issues was also the most common style that moms used to initiate discussions about sexuality. Estelle Brown, for instance, looked to events in the media and what was happening with Sam's peers to set the stage for delving into a particular topic.

One means of communicating that receives short shrift today, even though it continues to carry tremendous weight, is the age-old channel of unspoken messages. Girls spoke time and again about the messages conveyed by a mother's facial expression, by what was not said, and by what a mother did. Because many moms described with sadness that this was how they had "learned" from their own mothers, they did not, by and large, want to rely on the unspoken when it came to matters of sexuality. Still, these unspoken missives seem to be powerful today. Girls reported that they could tell "from the look on a [mother's] face" how she felt about an issue. Facial expressions, particularly when a girl saw disapproval in her mom's eyes or, as one put it, "that phony smile on her face," were dead giveaways.

It is not uncommon for a daughter to receive mixed messages from her mother's body language, however, particularly around sexual topics. Although moms try very hard to be open and honest with their daughters about sexual issues, it is inevitable that on some subjects a mother will feel unsure how to respond or ambivalent about her own feelings. She may say what she thinks she *should* say when she is really feeling something quite different. And the nonverbal message conveyed by a look or a frown can be the one that is most lasting. Ideally, if the mother can talk about her mixed feelings, her daughter will understand that the subject is one that doesn't lend itself to simple answers.

One girl noted that these unspoken messages ran both ways and that her mom had a sixth sense — "She just knows what's in my head." Others stated that a mother's own actions and attitudes about relationships had the greatest impact on their behavior. In the girls' minds, parents whose implicit messages were of the "do as I say not as I do" variety were not helpful.

The good news, then, is that mothers are communicating with their girls about sex and sexuality, and on some level their words — and gestures — carry weight. But both mothers and daughters also made clear how many external sources influence what girls know about sex and play into their decision-making processes. Mothers are not talking in a vacuum, and it is the broader context, the sometimes conflicting messages, that girls must sift through and synthesize to come to a larger understanding of sex and sexuality. Eventually, usually in midadolescence, they begin to look outside the family, perhaps for more detailed information they don't feel comfortable asking their mothers about. Where else are our girls learning about sex, sexuality, and sexual health? Though some of the sources are not surprising, the kinds and extent of information or misinformation these sources provide give cause for reflection.

## Peers

Katrina Shattuck identified the elements of sex best learned at home and those best learned from peers. In her estimation, "the basics should be learned at home, like, you know, where did you come from. I was a pretty curious child and I was always asking my mom questions. I had my ideas about the wedding ring doing something magical to make you a mother, but when I asked, my mom told me how it worked in kind of scientific terms. But when I got to school I learned a lot more and then I really understood what was going on."

Katrina revealed a trend among the older girls in the group, who were turning more often to their peers for information. "Later, from friends and my sister, I learned that there are varieties of sex. I don't think my mom could have told me that. And I learned about the bases, and, oh, I think to this day my mom doesn't know about the bases." Katrina explained what "the bases" meant to her and her friends: "First is frenching, second is being felt up, third is down the pants, and fourth is h-o-m-e-r-u-n. Then there are all the variations, like messy second and messy third, when a guy uses his mouth." The bases metaphor gave Katrina and her friends a shorthand for discussing information that otherwise made them feel awkward, but Katrina couldn't imagine discussing with her mom who was on which base. "It's embarrassing enough to talk about stuff with my sister and my close friends. I couldn't do that with mom."

Mothers and daughters agreed that girlfriends became an increasingly valuable source of sexual information as girls moved into midadolescence. Evelyn Shepherd commented, "Of course the peers are in-

evitable. They are always talking about 'it.'" Evelyn believed that discussions with friends could be valuable "if the kids have the right information." Estelle Brown thought that the most common source of
information for teens was their peers, as did Gerry Valentia. Alma
Parks wasn't convinced, however, about the quality of information that
girls were passing along to each other: "I can't say that talking to her
friends will help her; it might be a bad influence because a lot of messages they pass on today are not positive. They will make fun of a girl
who's a virgin."

Though many of the older girls spoke of their girlfriends as important providers of information, they also had some reservations about its
reliability — and about its believability. How much is handed over for
boasting privileges? Katrina, at fifteen, recalled her early adolescence:
"Anybody could ask you how far you got in any place. I remember
about ten kids asking me at the bus stop how far I had gotten with this
guy, and I was just mortified. I felt really pressured, so we were both
lying to other people about how far we had gone because if you didn't
do everything right away, you were a prude." By high school she had
found the confidence to step back and say, "It's not anyone's business."

Katrina's account draws attention to an overriding problem with
peer information: teens embellish, exaggerate, mischaracterize, and
even lie. As the teens in one of the focus groups noted, they learned
about sex "from friends, but we understand this information is inaccurate. . . . Friends exaggerate about sex." Though everyone was eager to
swap "locker room talk," the consensus was that you couldn't trust
what your classmates told you. Boys, it seemed, were more likely to
commit sins of commission and boast about their prowess, while girls
favored sins of omission.[3] Even fourteen-year-old Carmen Rankin,
generally cautious when dating, was surprised and angry when a boy
with whom she had petted bragged to his classmates that they had
"gone all the way."

A girl who thinks she is the only virgin in her class may begin to
wonder what's wrong with her, when, in fact, she may be one of the
few truth-tellers. On the other hand, girls who are sexually active may

keep silent with their friends. More than 40 percent of teens in one survey, both virgins and nonvirgins, thought their friends would "be shocked" if they told them they were having sexual intercourse.[4]

As we all know, peer pressure can bring enormous strife to young lives. The questions of whether to "do it," when to do it, how to do it are hard for teens to answer without taking into account the many different role models in their lives. While girls cited the importance of their mothers' words, we also know that peers' words carry tremendous weight. In one survey conducted by Planned Parenthood, adolescents reported that pressure from peers was, in fact, the most potent factor in their decision to become sexually active.[5]

Though parents have every right to worry about peer pressure, teenage girls can also provide wonderful support systems for each other, as Ruth Rosenbloom illustrated. "My friends and I, we talk most of the time. A lot of my friends, I could just talk to them the whole day and we wouldn't run out of things to say. We talk about our classes, what happened during the day, what the guys are like at school this year." It was at camp, though, she said, that the subject of sex came up most often, for summer friendships quickly fostered close confidences. "Some of the girls have already had sex and then some want to. Others are like me. You know, I'm going to wait. It's just too big of a thing to do now and regret it later."

Friends provided advice, and sometimes their experiences drove home lessons about sex that might not otherwise have registered so pointedly. Ruth, for instance, had been reunited with an old junior high friend who had been out of touch for some time. She recalled what a role model this girl had been: "She had a ninety-eight or more in all her classes. She was very smart and spoke two or three languages. And she had a boyfriend. I mean she was perfect." Yet now her friend was smoking and confessed that she might be pregnant because of a drunken one-night stand. Ruth's perfect image of her friend was shattered. "I still can't get over that she's so different. I don't know what happened."

Invaluable confidants, cherished sources of information, consultation, and consolation, girlfriends, when they venture off the beaten path, can also inspire confusion and pain. Ruth, at a loss to explain how her talented young friend could fall into self-destructive behavior, didn't know what she could to to provide support. Adolescence is characterized by teens' comparative judging: "I wouldn't ever do that" or "She's not a good person because she did such and such." Or "Well, if she's doing it, then maybe I should be doing it, too." Unfortunately, there's a good bit of self-judging as well: "If I did that, then I must not be a good person" or "If I am not doing that, there must be something wrong with me." Although teens may share with each other the immediacy and intensity of their feelings, they lack the broader perspective that we acquire over time to make sense of some of their more surprising actions.

Learning from one's peers is like working a jigsaw puzzle without the top to the box; girlfriends bring bits of information to the table, and the group pieces together what they think might be the correct picture. But they have no independent verification. This is normal and part of the fun of being a teen. Young people should be working out their own scripts, but often the script a young woman chooses for herself is influenced by the people with whom she associates. For someone like Erica, who had a difficult family situation and lived in a tough neighborhood, friends and her sixteen-year-old cousin were the only real positive role models in her life. Girls like Samantha, though, who are involved in community volunteering, sports, arts activities, Scouting, or other extracurricular opportunities, have more sources of information and a wider field of contacts in learning what to trust and what to disregard.

Parents cannot choose their children's friends — nor should they try — but they can suggest, nudge, and guide girls into activities that will engage both mind and body and provide a broader network of peer contacts and information.

## Media and Advertising

Many mothers, after citing the importance of peers, emphasized the heavy influence of television, movies, and videos on their children's knowledge of sexual activity. Emily Shattuck spoke for others when she explained that Katrina knew everything about sex — mostly from television and movies. Betty Graham had her own take on the media's influence on her daughter's sexual knowledge. "Television is the worst," she said. "Those people have no clue. I don't know what their motivations are, but it's certainly not part of our life — transvestites, sex crimes, all that deviant behavior."

Teens told a similar story. In the focus groups, adolescents stressed how much they learned from television. "We learn about sex from the soaps. They're doing it all the time on these shows," we heard. "TV, ads, and especially magazines encourage teens to think about being, acting or dressing sexy. From the talk shows we hear about what is forbidden."

Indeed, it would be very hard *not* to learn about sex from television. Three out of every four shows in the eight P.M. to nine P.M. slot, according to a recent survey, "contain sexually related talk or behavior." This is a fourfold increase from twenty years ago. And any parent who has watched any of the twelve most popular prime time programs for adolescents in recent years, shows like *The Fresh Prince of Bel Air, The Simpsons,* and *Beverly Hills 90210,* knows they contain abundant sexual references. A careful content analysis reveals just how abundant: "On average, 29 percent of the interactions on an individual episode of these shows contained verbal references to sexual issues, with the level surpassing 50 percent for some episodes." Messages about male sexual roles in these shows outnumbered those about female sexual roles, and when sex was covered, the emphasis was on its recreational aspect rather than on procreation. In the most frequent messages, sexual relationships were depicted as competitions, men commented on women's bodies and physical appearance, and loving and respectful relationships were downplayed.[6]

A closer look at the six most popular shows among adolescents in 1995 for messages about sex and interactions with sexual content drives the point home: for *The Fresh Prince of Bel Air,* ranking number one among teens, 38 percent of interactions had sexual content; for *Blossom,*

59 percent; *Roseanne* had 32 percent; *Martin,* 49 percent; *The Simpsons,* 19 percent; and *Beverly Hills 90210,* 28 percent.[7]

When sex is depicted on television, it is usually "without consequence, without worry, and with rarely a bad experience." Soap operas seem to be the "worst offenders." As a recent report put it, "Sex is frequently portrayed as being impersonal and exploitative, birth control is rarely mentioned, and sex between unmarried partners is 24 times more common [on soap operas] than sex between spouses." One group of researchers found that girls who are just beginning to gain sexual and romantic experience are especially fascinated by the media's depiction of male-female relationships.[8]

Noting the prevalence of sex on television and establishing its influence on teens and their actions are two different matters, of course. Yet some powerful lessons can be learned from broader surveys. In one study conducted a few years ago at the University of New Mexico, researchers examined how much time the average child between the ages of two and eighteen spends watching television, how she or he learns from television, and how television influences attitudes and behaviors, including aggressiveness and sexuality. The findings revealed that, on average, American youngsters are exposed annually to more than 14,000 sexual references, innuendoes, and jokes. Less than 175 of these images deal with birth control, abstinence, or sexually transmitted diseases. The report warned: "Unfortunately, young people are getting more unhealthy information than healthy information from the media. When sex is used to sell everything from cars to shampoo and human sexuality is displayed irresponsibly, children and adolescents derive important cues about adult behavior."[9]

Such statistics can quickly take on real meaning at home. One night, for example, Joan Rankin watched one of Carmen's favorite TV shows, *Beverly Hills 90210,* with her daughter. In this episode the lead girl, Brenda, has sex with her boyfriend on prom night. "The couple is going into this hotel room looking all lovey-dovey," Joan said. "Later they come out and look really happy." After the program Carmen asked nonchalantly, "Oh, is that what it's like?" Joan felt compelled to give her a dose of reality. "Not always," she said. "I'm surprised that they didn't show her [the girl] to be a little uncomfortable because often, for the first time, sexual intercourse is really painful." Joan told Carmen she didn't think it was realistic when all the girlfriends congratulated Brenda, and she didn't believe that the parents' reaction to the girl's subsequent fear that she might be pregnant rang true. "They were just too unconcerned, I told her."

In my interview with Carmen, she mentioned the same show and ended her recounting of the conversation with, "When my mom explained all that to me, I was really shocked." Had Joan not had this discussion with Carmen after the show, Carmen's expectations for "the first time" might have been sorely off base. Here was an example of using the media as a springboard for helpful conversation.

Movies amplify many of the sexual messages portrayed on television, and some scenes can make a parent's heart stop. "What television suggests, movies and videos do," observed one media analyst.[10] Explicit sex in the movies is about as prevalent as popcorn, and formerly taboo topics are now presented in Panavision with Surroundsound. Both parents and teens laughed about the movie rating systems. "Keeping teens out of R-rated movies might work at a few theaters," one parent said, "but it doesn't make any difference. My kids can go down to the video store and rent any movie they want any time of the day."

The authors of *Mother-Daughter Revolution: From Betrayal to Power* point out that girls are introduced to sexuality early on through children's romance stories and even fairy tales projected on the screen. In the guise of romance, the authors assert, "Disney's *Aladdin* shows girls that by lying and trading sexual favors, they can get what they want. *Beauty and the Beast* gives girls the dubious message that 'true love' can transform a beast into a prince."[11] And for teens, much more explicit movie messages abound. In the ever-popular *Pretty Woman*, for instance, we learn that if the prostitute is pretty and charming enough, the rich and dashing hero marries her. "The romance plot line shapes girls' understanding of their own experience. Good girls have sex when it is 'true love.' "

We lack definitive answers as to how and in what ways our adolescents are being influenced by television and other media sources on sexuality. But those who have looked into the matter tell us we can at least answer the question "Is it having an effect on our children?" with a qualified "Yes." As the teens in the MCC groups explained, their attitudes about sex often came from what was on the television screen.[12]

Different teens, of course, will process these electronic messages in different ways. Tiffany Henderson reassured her mom, "I'm fifteen years old and I've seen a lot of stuff in movies and on television and I've been fine up until now. Just because they do something on TV doesn't mean I'm dumb enough to go out and do it too." Samantha, two years older, had also learned that life as portrayed on television didn't necessarily mesh with the real world. "Kids are going to learn a lot from peers and the media," she said, "but a lot of this stuff is false — you're getting false outlooks. It's like you should have sex with every person you go out with and it's not a special thing; it's just something you're supposed to do." She was amazed by the rosy glasses through which the media portrayed sex: "Nothing ever happens," Sam said. "You can't get hurt by having sex and things like that, and I know it isn't true because my friend got pregnant and her boyfriend just left her."

Another pervasive influence is rock music. The lyrics range from "Come over to my house so we can do it" to "Let's not rush into it." As one girl commented in an interview on the influence of media, "The guy in the song who was talking about sex as being good seemed happy. Janet [Jackson] sounded sad and depressed. I really know which is the right way, but sometimes, the way the media talks about it, you really begin to wonder."[13]

Don't parents have a right to be concerned, even angry, about the messages their daughters are receiving from the media? Newton Minow, the former chairman of the Federal Communications Commission, raged that "no other major democratic nation in the world has so willingly turned its children over to mercenary strangers the way we have with television and movies. . . . Psychologists and social scientists know that this system does measurable harm and that used wisely, television could do measurable good."[14]

In fact, television producers have made some strides in emphasizing the importance of loving and caring relationships and also responsible sexual behavior. On one episode of *Blossom,* for example, a group of teens created a sex video with a script that read, "Don't be ashamed to carry a condom. It doesn't mean you're going to have sex. It just means you're prepared if you do." And *Beverly Hills 90201* aired an episode in which a young woman on her way into a bedroom stopped at the restroom to get a condom, saying, "Better safe than sorry." And *Party of Five* dealt sensitively with a young woman's dilemma about whether or not to have an abortion. Such episodes tell teens that sexual and romantic relationships are not always carefree, that they always involve responsibility and sometimes pain and conflict.[15]

What have not changed in television and movies, however, are the very traditional portrayals of men and women. Female characters tend to worry about looking attractive, about the shapes of their bodies and seduction strategies, while men focus on how successful they are at "scoring."[16] This trend extends to advertising in our neighborhoods, on our billboards, and in our mail as well. Advertisers bank on the beauty message to resonate for girls, and its connection to sexual appeal is seldom far behind. Sex is used to sell everything.

Thin, pretty girls have always been used as a strong marketing tool. Yet even to a casual observer, the ads in recent years have become more suggestive and sexual. Consider the Levi's poster that stopped me cold when I saw it plastered to my neighborhood bus stop. A teenage girl sitting in a boy's lap faces her partner with her legs spread apart, leaving the viewer to speculate on whose zipper is up or down. It is not the durability, versatility, or popularity of the Levi's jeans that this ad stresses, but the sexiness of the people in them.

Copious sexual images fill the pages of magazines and cyberspace, and while their tenor has become more explicit, many a mother feels we've grown rather resigned to it. "I remember," says one middle-aged woman with grown children, "my parents' hiding my father's *Esquire* magazine with the pinup centerfold. And I remember finding a girlie magazine hidden under my son's bed. Now the *Victoria's Secret* catalogue comes in the mail, and it's more risqué than any centerfold I remember from those days." The teens we talked with in focus groups were clear about the influence of advertising. Ads in magazines, they told us, "encourage teens to think about being sexy, acting sexy, and dressing sexy."[17]

In addition, some teen magazines deliver cross-messages to girls in their articles and their advertising. An inspection of the editorial and advertising content of teen magazines for girls published during a three-year period, for instance, revealed that though the advice column recommended that girls postpone sex, the advertising displays encouraged them to become sexual objects.[18] And a study of approximately 4,000 network television commercials found that one of every 3.8 commercials included some type of attractiveness-based message. "Although most ads don't directly model sexual intercourse," the authors wrote, "they help set the stage for sexual behavior by promoting the importance of beautiful bodies and products that enhance attractiveness. Advertisers like Calvin Klein, Guess jeans, Levi's, and Benetton have pushed the limits of sexual suggestiveness with their use of bared flesh, childlike models, and intertwined limbs."[19] Advertisers would not spend millions of dollars on the images they present if they did not unequivocally believe the old adage "a picture is worth a thousand words."

There are, thankfully, many other visual resources for our girls, including books that relay thoughtful and careful information about sex and sexuality. Oddly, though, with the exception of Ingrid and one other girl who had taken a sexually explicit book to her Catholic school (much to the nuns' dismay), none of the girls mentioned books or magazines as a primary source of information. When books came up in the conversation, it was more often by mothers, who recalled their own moms handing them a book as their complete "sex education." One woman recalled her grandmother's lending her a medical textbook filled with anatomical drawings, including misshapen and diseased penises. She was terrified of anything having to do with sex after glimpsing those pictures. Happily, there are many more well-done, developmentally appropriate books today that do a thorough job of explaining issues of sexuality.

Recently there has also been an explosion of creative information for girls — in video games, on the Internet, and in print media — that goes way beyond thin and sexy to challenge female sexual stereotypes. The comic book *Get Real* featured in its first issue women of all colors collaborating, girls playing soccer, and boys baby-sitting. Other new magazines, such as *Jump*, which bills itself as the publication "for girls who dare to be real," and *Blue Jeans*, which promotes itself as a publication that has no beauty tips, fashion spreads, or supermodels, offer important alternatives for adolescent girls.[20]

Such alternative publications are a welcome addition to the teen magazine scene, especially since in the past mainstream publications have been limited in their ability to speak forthrightly to girls. When *Sassy*, a popular publication aimed at teenage girls, first appeared, its editor wrote of her commitment to providing teens with "responsible, direct information about sex," and both teens and parents responded appreciatively. But when articles like "Losing Your Virginity," "Getting Turned On," and "My Girlfriend Got Pregnant" appeared, the religious right was outraged and organized an advertisers' boycott.[21] Although these articles were meant to educate and inform teenagers, not sell them on the benefits of early sex, *Sassy* gave in to political pressure and removed material that acknowledged and addressed adolescent desire.

## Within Jefferson's and Nottingham's Classrooms

When Katrina Shattuck said, "I've learned a heck of a lot in school about sexual stuff," she spoke for many of the Nottingham girls. In fact, three-fourths of the girls in my research groups mentioned school as a source for their sexual knowledge. With the exception of Joan Rankin, all of the mothers and daughters agreed it was important for schools to include sex education in their curriculums. At both public and private school, most girls mentioned having had their first personal-growth class around fifth grade, where they received instruction about conception and watched a film on menstruation.

Jefferson girls enjoyed their ninth-grade personal-growth class, while Nottingham teens said their growth-education classes, beginning in seventh grade and continuing through tenth, contributed a great deal to their sexual knowledge. Overall the classes had been positive experiences for the girls, and many said that they were allowed to speak in the classroom on topics, such as contraception, that they wouldn't have felt comfortable discussing at home. Angela and Samantha both spoke of how helpful it was to have teachers who were sensitive and comfortable talking about sex. Classes sometimes evolved into free-wheeling question-and-answer sessions in which kids threw out their wildest questions. Bettina described how in her seventh-grade personal-growth class, everyone would start to giggle at the mention of reproduction, but by eighth grade the tenor of the conversation had turned: "We started talking about relationships and everyone has been a little more serious." Tiffany Henderson was another who felt the classes enhanced her knowledge and understanding of sexual issues, since "parents can't always tell you everything [and] . . . may not be as blunt as someone who doesn't know you that well." She was glad to have seen different birth control products at school.

Mothers were generally very supportive of their children's participation in these classes. In fact, the teachers of personal-growth classes at both schools noted that over the several years they had been teaching, they could each recall only one parent who had requested that a child be exempted. The teachers at both schools worked to get parents' support as well. Nottingham, for instance, offered an orientation session for all seventh-grade parents that outlined the course curriculum.

Marian Henderson and Gerry Valentia were very comfortable with the material being taught at their respective schools, though they stressed the importance of providing kids with some sort of moral context at home. "Children," Marian explained, "need to be taught their values at home." Gerry was grateful that the classes prompted conversations with Carolyn at home. "Sure, I sometimes feel ambivalent,"

Gerry confessed, "when I hear about some of the topics they discuss at school, but I always wanted my children to participate in these programs."

Joan Rankin, however, did not want her child involved in any class that addressed sexuality. Having taught a sex education class in a parochial school herself, Joan was uncomfortable with what she saw as the public school classes' lack of emphasis on values. "I heard how they sensationalize sex and give the message that you can do whatever you like," she said. "It's just 'Here, have a condom and don't worry about it.'" When Carmen's science class compiled a list of all the slang terms students knew for penis and vagina, Joan was furious. "I do think sex education should be taught in school, but it should be taught in a matter-of-fact way within a moral context," she said.

As a private school, Nottingham had much more flexibility in what it could incorporate in its personal-growth classes, which each year focused on particular topics. Seventh-graders discussed values, friendship, self-esteem, cultural stereotypes, sexual harassment, family relationships, communication, and AIDS. Sexuality and puberty were also introduced.

In Nottingham's eighth-grade class, the mechanics of reproduction were reviewed, and students began to learn about abstinence, birth control, and preventable sexual health problems. By ninth grade, students focused more on the emotional and psychological components of relationships. In tenth grade, the class became primarily student-led: teams of two researched a topic and presented their findings to the class.

At Jefferson, ninth-graders counted on the teacher, Mrs. Mackey, to give them straight answers when they asked tough questions. As she explained her own goals, the emphasis in her class was "on her students' understanding the changes that are taking place in their bodies and on developing decision-making skills." Her course emphasized the importance of abstinence but also covered contraception for protection against pregnancy and disease. Mrs. Mackey sometimes questioned "whether what I'm doing makes much of an impact. . . . I'll think they have their heads screwed on right, but when I see that we have two hundred students in our parenting programs at Jefferson, I wonder." Still, she was pleased when her graduates returned to tell her how important her class had been to them.

It is heartening to know that the girls at Nottingham and Jefferson were getting useful advice in their sex education classes, but teens across America tell us they still aren't receiving enough information in the classroom. In a recent Kaiser Foundation survey of 1,510 youths, ages twelve to eighteen, the majority wanted more practical information about sexuality, including facts on how to get and use birth control before they became sexually involved. These adolescents also said they looked mostly to teachers, school nurses, and sex education classes for contraceptive information. While 74 percent had talked with at least one of their parents about sex, only 46 percent said they had talked specifically about birth control. Some 55 percent had discussed sexually transmitted diseases with their parents. Schools and the country need to respond to the 95 percent of the students in the Kaiser survey who stated that when they did get information about birth control it came too late and didn't include enough detail.[22]

## Words from on High

One Saturday Evelyn Shepherd took Ingrid for a haircut. The stylist chatted with Ingrid about school and boys. Suddenly she stopped trimming and said to Ingrid, "I've just got two things to say to you. You stay in school and finish up your education, and you don't go messing around with sex till you're married, and even then, you don't mess." Ingrid's mouth flew open — she was speechless. Evelyn couldn't believe that her daughter's hairdresser was delivering a morality message that no one in the Shepherds' church — or school, as far as she knew — had ever come close to articulating. "This is what I meant," Evelyn explained to me, "when I talked to you about the failure of institutions."

A few mothers looked to their religious institutions for guidance concerning sex and sexuality. The Rankins were prepared to follow the teachings of the Catholic church, and Rebecca Tate, who favored "holding to the old-time ways," relied on her Pentecostal religion for sexual values. But the remainder of the mothers and daughters, whether Protestant, Catholic, Jewish, or of another faith, said that their religious institutions had little to say about sexuality. Julie King and Mary Robbins, in particular, expressed frustration with the church's silence on teen pregnancy, when it was so obviously a problem for some of its young parishioners.

Girls like Ruth Rosenbloom were also aware of this hushed silence: "No one from temple has said much about sexuality. Religion doesn't really play a role in how I will make those decisions." Carolyn Valentia, who had gone to Catholic elementary school, said she retained many of the church's values but with her own modifications; if she became sexually active, she explained, she would not herself use contraception but would insist that her partner use a condom. This interesting twist of interpretation allowed her to honor the church's teachings while still protecting herself. Girls in the focus groups, when asked what influenced their thoughts and decisions about becoming sexually active, reported overwhelmingly, "No influence from the church."

Some mothers followed the advice of my favorite aunt: "Never let the teachings of the church get in the way of your faith." If the churches these women belonged to opposed contraception, they advised their daughters to take the rule "with a grain of salt." Their faith in God should not keep them from protecting themselves sexually.

Girls who receive a consistent and unambiguous message from both church and home that there will be no sex before marriage, no birth control, and no acceptance of homosexuality or abortion have the clear advantage of an authoritative stance from adults. Such a stance can be helpful as they work out their ethical dilemmas, for they know exactly what they are bouncing up against and can then accept or reject the rules. But this kind of clarity can bring its own difficulties. The lack of ambiguity can make any failure to observe the tenets of the church particularly shameful. And it can, if girls are not careful, foster intolerance and judgmental attitudes.

Considered together, sex and religion may be even more of a hot potato than sex and schools. Many leaders of religious institutions are uneasy discussing the topic. They either say little about it or present their positions in a form so simplified — and sometimes so rigid — that they may fail to reach their teenager members and, in many cases, the parents of these teens. Parents like Evelyn Shepherd and Mary Robbins wanted more guidance from their churches. Schools could provide a sound factual basis and a place for helpful peer dialogue, but they expected religious leaders to help their daughters place the sexual facts in a moral framework. When the church failed, they had to turn elsewhere — even to someone as unlikely as the neighborhood hairdresser.

## New Community Resources

If schools are tentative and religious institutions reluctant or rigid in addressing teen sexuality, other community institutions are making advances. Girls Incorporated, a national organization that has adopted as its mission "to take a leadership role as an advocate for the rights and needs of girls of all backgrounds and abilities," has developed an education program for girls from nine to eighteen that takes a comprehensive approach to teenage pregnancy prevention. Beginning with "Growing Together," a series of workshops for nine- to eleven-year-olds, it is designed to foster positive communication between parents and daughters about sexual information and values. The second phase, aimed at girls twelve to fourteen, "Will Power/Won't Power," encourages early adolescents to delay sexual intercourse. The third phase, "Taking Care of Business," aims to help girls fifteen to eighteen increase their educational and career planning skills as well as their motivation to avoid pregnancy. A final component, "Health Bridge," links educational opportunities available in local Girls Clubs with community-based health services.[23]

Responding to the same needs, the federal Department of Health and Human Services (HHS) recently launched a national public education campaign called "Girl Power!," aimed at nine- to fourteen-year-old girls. The campaign will focus on motivating parents, schools, religious groups, health care providers, and community groups to reinforce girls' self-confidence with positive opportunities and accurate information on key health issues.[24]

The most active national group today helping girls address issues related to sexuality is Planned Parenthood. Beyond providing health services, this organization, which has more than 168 affiliates nationwide, offers many mother-daughter workshops and reaches out to more than 1.5 million people each year. In fact, three-quarters of Planned Parenthood's work consists of training professionals in community organizations, who then deliver local sexuality education programs. In St. Paul, Minnesota, for instance, mothers and their young daughters can be part of a program called "Making the Connection — A Day of Discovery for Mothers and Daughters," which incorporates wilderness activities with relationship building and sexuality issues. In Lubbock, Texas, mothers with daughters between ages ten and fifteen can sign up for "Mothers — Let's Talk," a program that focuses on communication about body changes, puberty, self-esteem, and self-defense.[25]

Katrina Shattuck and other members of her family may have found it far easier to deal with some of the questions and issues surrounding her sister's sexual orientation if they had known of a community organization that provided such support. Now, in a number of cities, gay and lesbian community centers provide a range of sources. Some have hot lines and pen-pal programs for young people who have questions about their sexual orientation or who, like Katrina, just need someone who will listen and understand what they're dealing with. Another group, Parents and Friends of Lesbian and Gays (PFLAG), offers chapters in many cities that meet regularly to provide support, counseling, and other services to parents of gay and lesbian children.[26]

## Using Our Resources

Although we seem to have numerous sources of information for teens to tap into on adolescent topics, there is a reluctance in our culture to provide them with the facts they need about sexual topics. Perhaps we confuse facts with feeling. We seem to believe that if we make sexual information more available, we will encourage teens to have sex. But I have concluded, from the years I have spent in this work, that if we were more forthcoming about the facts, our messages about feelings would be better heard. If sexual topics were less political, less dangerous to discuss and debate, we would not be so caught up in the controversies over whether to say this word or advertise that product, and we could move the focus from sex to relationships.

All of the sources mentioned in this chapter can add valuable voices, wisdom, and perspectives to mothers' conversations with their daughters. I believe that those who advocate keeping sex education in the home have misplaced the emphasis. Let our schools or girls' clubs display the anatomical charts, show slides of the reproductive system, pass around various methods of contraception, and define, as with any other vocabulary word, homosexuality, masturbation, bestiality, testosterone, menses, pubic, clitoris, and so on. Let them create a safe space in which adolescents can talk with one another about the issues. Then parents can lend even more emphasis to such important topics as equality in a relationship, values, the characteristics of maturity in a partnership, and their hopes for their girls and for their daughters' future children.

# SIX

# With an Eye
# to the Future

...................❖....................

**K**it, an energetic, ponytailed girl just starting high school, was talking with her three best friends about what they valued in a relationship with a boy. "I'm big on love," Kit said. "What I really think about all the time is how much I want my own true love because I think love brings happiness." Her best friend demurred. "Me, I'm not ready for love. I think I'm too young. I just want to be touched." Honor-roll students, class leaders, and athletes in their schools, these girls passed endless hours talking together about boys. "You know, we spend a lot of time figuring out how to position ourselves; how to stand and what we'll say; when we're going to do what and what he might do, and all that stuff."

Talking with a boy, they explained, can make a girl feel better than anything else. "If a guy calls and you talk, when you get off the phone, you feel so giddy and happy. You want to just jump on your bed. It gives you a boost in confidence." But even better than that, they confessed, was being touched. "Messing around, making out, it just makes you feel . . . you know, alive." Touching took them beyond the limits of their good-girl lives to something more exciting, more risky, less controlled, and they coveted that excitement. "But it's funny," one of the girls conceded. "We say we want a boyfriend, and then we really don't because the boys aren't that interesting. It's the chase we like."

And then there is the talking. The girls loved the hours of stretching out on each other's beds and swapping fantasies, comparing strategies and sharing gossip. "I just like my friends," Cindy explained. "We talk about everything. I don't know what I'd be doing without my friends." Any topic was fair game, from masturbation to breast size, from petting to party clothes. "Sometimes we just take off our shirts and compare our breasts," Kit said.

These girls were reveling in the preciousness of adolescent friendship, at that age when friends become one's closest confidants. But even when talking about "positioning" themselves for boys, they didn't appear to be transforming themselves to please their young Romeos. Rather, their words bespoke the adventure and excitement of trying to gain a boy's admiration — and the fun of trading stories with friends. Pursuing a serious relationship could be nice, but in the end, compared to themselves, boys weren't all that captivating. Kit and her friends were striking that balance between wanting to feel alive and not eclipsing their own sense of self-worth.

## Striving for a Sense of Self

For the girls at Jefferson and Nottingham, searching for love and acceptance while maintaining their self-confidence was a juggling act they performed each day. Some seemed to pull it off with the aplomb of Kit and her friends, while for others it was a herculean task. It's easy to think that adolescent girls' only passions lie in the right sneaker brand, mall cruising, boys, and call waiting. Those amusements were certainly part of their lives, but they were also struggling to figure out who they wanted to be, in school, in their future careers, in their adult lives. Looking back on our talks, I was amazed at the extent to which they were weighing their sexuality and their potential and current relationships in a much broader context. The girls spoke generally of their personal aspirations, worries, and concerns for the people they loved.

The desire to be thought of in a positive light by peers and others creates tension for just about every teenager, but it shows itself in different guises. The older girls in my group looked forward to boys' attention. They wanted to feel comfortable with their emerging sexual desire but were wary of being tagged as a "slut" if their friends thought they were flirting too openly or "coming on" to a boy. They grasped all too well the threats to their reputations posed by innuendoes and gossip, and they carefully guarded those reputations. But beyond seeking acceptance as bona fide members of their peer groups, they emphasized how important it was for their parents to like them, to be proud of their school performance, and to approve of their social selves. The conversations of both Nottingham and Jefferson girls often alluded to wanting to do right by those who were raising them.

Trying to please everyone, though, including themselves, was not always easy. Achieving that balance in their everyday family, school, and social lives posed a challenge for more than a few. Fourteen-year-old Cindy Gordon, for instance, expressed her strong will when she talked about how hard it was to make decisions: "It's hard not to do what others want you to, even when you know it isn't the right thing for yourself." Cindy's friends liked "to drink and get wasted" on the weekends. "I'd rather stay conscious," she said. "But it's difficult when a lot of people say to you, 'You don't drink?'" For Cindy, trying to figure out what she wanted for herself and how much others' choices would sway her decisions presented a conflict most weekends. Lately she had found that everyone else disagreed with her position on drinking.

She also worried about getting a bad reputation and disappointing her parents if she did something considered "slutty." But she was at a loss to define what that meant. Some of her friends seemed to think a girl deserved to be called a slut if she had sex before she was fifteen, but Cindy sensed that "older people" had a broader definition of the term.

Fifteen-year-old Tiffany empathized with Cindy's struggles: "Between the ages of twelve and thirteen, I had a real problem with trying to do what people wanted me to do. Now I do what I have to do and have stopped worrying about all those other unimportant things. I need to stay true to myself." At fourteen, Erica, living with her aunt, from whom she felt emotionally detached, said that she had no choice but to take care of herself. "I'm not depending on anyone because I'm for me. I'm my own person. I have to make my choices and understand how life works."

Some of these girls, such as Erica and Anita, had been forced to grow up quickly, but no matter what their age, they were all addressing the conflicting pressures of adolescence. While Ruth talked about how invaluable her friends were and how much more she now, at fifteen, turned to them for advice, she, too, was striving to define her own limits. She spoke poignantly of a friend whom she thought had been overwhelmed by her desire to be accepted by peers: "I think, actually, that she stopped being able to be sure of herself. . . . She wanted to be liked by these new friends, and it just got worse and worse. She was trying to be like who she really wasn't." Ruth concluded, "I don't think you can do that in high school or even in college. Being a follower doesn't work; you can talk to your friends about certain things. I go to them about some problems, but I really need to make decisions for myself."

Those who followed their own passions in extracurricular activities at school seemed to be doing a good job of juggling adolescent stresses. Carolyn, whose self-esteem had grown remarkably, told any boy she went out with that he had to understand that her "friends come first, then basketball, and then you." Angela Parks, who could hold a room with her charisma and self-possession, was another whose self-esteem had been enhanced by her various roles at Jefferson. When I asked, for instance, what first came to mind when she thought of herself as a teenager, she replied, "Leader." She loved being with her friends but enjoyed reading books just as much. She also liked to write and confessed that she recorded her romantic fantasies in her journal.

The girls' voices were compassionate, insightful, funny, futuristic, and hopeful. The concerns closest to their hearts were family members and friends, school success, keeping themselves and others out of harm's way, becoming emotionally and, someday, economically independent, and being thought of as a good person in all of their relationships.

## Living Up to Expectations

There are enormous pressures on girls today to live up to parents' expectations. Though it may seem that teens do everything in their power to push our buttons, those I spoke with were sometimes obsessed with trying to please their parents as well as their teachers and friends. For girls at Nottingham, in particular, school performance was a source of urgent worry. They were constantly anxious about being able to meet the academic standards and expectations set for them by parents and teachers. Those who were already aware of the requirements for competitive colleges and graduate schools worried about their grade-point averages and the Scholastic Achievement Tests (SATs) they would have to take later in high school. When they pushed these worries aside, parents and teachers offered reminders and admonitions about the importance of excelling in their academic work. For fifteen-year-old Nicole Lee, the pressure to excel in school sometimes brought about physical distress. She would develop migraines or become sick to her stomach just thinking about her grades. "If I get anything below a B, I get scared. I get so stressed out and afraid of what my parents will do that it distracts me, so I end up with B+ and A− work. Sometimes when I just forget about it, I do better work." In dance Nicole had found a welcome release: "Dancing takes me away from it, because no one can get at you. . . . There I'm safe."

Tiffany had become more studious, but she agonized that colleges might not accept her, thus diminishing her shot at the career she wanted. "When I was younger I used to say I was going to go to the best college and get the best job," she reflected. "Now as I get closer to it, I'm like, hey, it's not that easy. There are a lot of people that I'm competing against who are really good and sometimes I just want to say, 'Forget it,' and then I say, 'No, no.' I just have to keep egging my-self on." Contemplating two more years of high school, four years of college, and then graduate school, Tiffany groaned, "It seems like a long time. I think sometimes I'm going to wake up and it's all going to be over my head."

Despite the anticipated long haul, for the most part the girls from both schools outlined their long-term goals, often echoing their moth-ers' dreams for them and often mixing determination with a dose of naiveté. Most envisioned themselves in school for several years beyond high school and set their sights on professional degrees. Jenny King, the thirteen-year-old from Nottingham, described her goals this way: "I want to be a successful lawyer and be a partner in my dad's law firm. . . . When I am twenty-five, I'll probably be working toward being accepted into the bar. I'll probably be toward the end of school or working in my dad's firm . . . climbing the corporate ladder." Ingrid, at fourteen, wanted first to be taller, but beyond that she aspired to be a writer. Fourteen-year-old Carmen, quiet and restrained in our meet-ing, outlined the following plan with gusto: "I want to go to college and go into political science and law. I want to be a lawyer and a politician and be the first woman president of the United States. . . . I really want to devote my life to a career."

One high school freshman who understood the importance of a career was overwhelmed by figuring out what was right for her. She confessed, "I've really, really thought about what I want to be, and I'm worried that time will run out — and I won't know."

In general, the girls possessed a great awareness of the importance and utility of education, much more so than high school girls of my generation. "I want to be independent. I'd like to be able to support myself in case something happens," Samantha said. With disarming pragmatism, she talked about the possibility of divorce and economic difficulties in her unfolding life. While she might have secretly been hoping for a happily-ever-after story line for herself, she and her girl-friends knew they couldn't bank on it. They had seen firsthand their parents or friends' parents go through divorce, and the Jefferson girls, in particular, understood the painful anxieties brought about by too little family income. When mothers emphasized the importance of financial independence, daughters got the message. "My mother," Tiffany said, "wants to make sure that everything goes right for me and that when I get old enough I will have a good background and I can set up things for myself, and I don't have to depend on anyone."

When the talk turned to their own future families, a few stated they did not want children, others were unsure, and still others wanted to "have a few kids." In speaking of relationships generally, the girls stressed mutual respect, care, and love. The majority reported that they might be involved in a caring and loving relationship with a boy by the end of high school, though Carolyn suspected she wouldn't have time to fall in love until she was about forty, given her basketball plans. The girls who were most adamant about wanting children seemed to be those from the worst family situations. For example, Tina, who had suffered abuse as a child, was the most enthusiastic about getting married and having a family. This is not an uncommon response for abused teens, who often are searching for someone to love them unconditionally.[1]

Still, Tiffany represented the majority opinion when she said, "I want to get a good education, go to college, get a good job, do something for other people and one day have a family. After everything is done, I may get married and have a kid or two." Like Katrina, who thought "absolutely, definitely" she would regret it if she didn't have a family "later in life," these girls were focusing on their independent selves first.

One difference did arise in their conversations regarding education, however. All of the girls at Nottingham assumed they would go on to college and even graduate school. It was expected of them — almost a rite of passage. Most of the girls from Jefferson were also thinking about graduate school, but their reasons subtly differed from those of the Nottingham girls. For those at Jefferson, higher education was seen not so much as life's normal course but as the ticket out of their current environment.

## Economic Uncertainty

Although both Jefferson and Nottingham girls had ambitious career aspirations, the Jefferson teens faced tougher economic challenges. Studies that have considered the effects of poverty on children underscore just how difficult it is for young women in circumstances like Erica's or Tina's to negotiate the many steps to success. It is hard enough for girls with supportive families and economic stability to chart a course that balances marriage, children, work, and self, but for those without economic support and role models, the task is even tougher. Today's young women are embarking on a life radically different from the status quo of earlier generations, when many mothers were schooling their daughters on how to land a good man to provide for them and their family. In the 1990s this formula rarely works (and it didn't always succeed a generation ago!). Girls with minimal education and limited job skills are especially at risk for becoming single young mothers living in poverty.

As Kristin Luker points out in her book *Dubious Conceptions*, on teenage pregnancy, "Dreams die hard." Most of the girls at Jefferson cited their ambitions to continue their education and have a career as well as a family. And why shouldn't they? None with whom I spoke, despite difficult financial circumstances now, wanted to end up as an unmarried mother on welfare, as the media might have us believe. "Many disadvantaged teens," Luker notes, "do dream of motherhood, they dream of white picket fence motherhood, or at least the version of it to which girls from poor neighborhoods can realistically aspire. . . . It's hard for people who have grown up in poverty to figure out how to make their dreams come true. . . . Young women of all classes must find a way to balance investments in their own future with commitment to a partner."[2]

I thought of Tina Watts, who spoke dreamily of finishing high school, going to college, getting married, and having children. Though her aunt was committed to doing everything in her power to help Tina achieve her goals, I wondered how a sixty-year-old single woman with a chronic illness and limited income would be able to support these endeavors. Moreover, in this time of increasing opportunities for women in general, opportunities for disadvantaged girls are in fact decreasing. As social historian Lisbeth Schorr points out, "Earlier in this century the routes up and out of poverty were imperfect, and they worked less well for blacks than for whites, but they were plentiful. . . . Today, escape has become harder and happens less often." More than a few of the girls I spoke with were unrealistic about how difficult it would be to make their way out of a disadvantaged environment.[3]

Still, for girls at Jefferson, ambition and education were the calling cards to a better life. Seeing the determination and dedication of these mothers and daughters, who were working and striving for more, I believed they had a good shot at beating some of these tremendous odds. As Angela Parks described her intentions, "I really want to be *known* — not famous, but I want to make a big mark . . . I want to change the world in a big way." I had little doubt that she would.

## Keep Me Safe

When the conversation switched from hopes to worries, all of the girls mentioned first their fears of imminent death or disaster. For some, death was a serious worry; in fact, for Jefferson students, violence and death were daily threats. Erica, who lived in one of her city's roughest neighborhoods, knew that a cavalier attitude toward safety could cost her her life. Her primary worry was that her twelve-year-old sister would be raped. Even feisty Angela, who also lived in a neighborhood lorded over by gangs, admitted, "Death, that's my biggest fear. . . . I don't want to die with pain. . . . I don't want to go before my time. I could go right out after this interview and never be seen again." More than one of the Jefferson girls delivered this same sentiment.

But Kit and two of her best friends, who lived in affluent urban neighborhoods, shared Erica's fear of being raped. "I worry about it all the time," Kit confessed. "There was this incident with the lifeguard at the pool. He told me to come into the back room, and then he started telling me what he was going to do to me, and even though I ran away and the police came, it still scared me." When another friend said she never thought about rape, her friend Tamara turned and said with exasperation, "That's why we have to think about it all the time, because we have to be scared for you."

Anita Dodson, fifteen and very striking, spoke of walking home from a party one night. Though she was supposed to leave with her sister, the sister wasn't ready to go, so Anita left on her own. "I saw this guy I sort of knew. He was about twenty-four and he had been drinking. He started walking and talking with me, and then he just grabbed me and pulled me into a vacant place off the sidewalk. I was kicking and hitting him with my pocketbook. I wasn't having any of that," she said. "He started trying to calm me down, and then he began to choke me and pull out his . . . About that time, I heard a friend call out, 'Anita, is that you?' When he heard her coming, he just grabbed my pocketbook and left. He threw my pocketbook down afterward, but he took all the money."

When Anita told her mother, they called the police. But according to Anita, the police did little to help. "They acted like they didn't care. I was really mad — mad at him because he tried to do that and mad at the police. Later I saw him, and he tried to apologize. But I said, 'It's too late.' " She trailed off. "He's in jail now."

Anita's ordeal was a haunting story for any mother or daughter to hear. Anita escaped physical harm, but two of the girls in my study did report having been raped, one by a friend of the family, another by her stepfather. One girl was able to come away from the ordeal determined that she would never be taken advantage of by anyone again, perhaps easier said than done. I sensed that the rape had influenced her attitudes toward sex; she told me she wanted to have sex to find out what it felt like when it was a *good* thing. Another girl was less fortunate; hungry for love, she was disturbingly willing to acquiesce to boys who promised the reward of sex. Rape was not just an ethereal fear for these girls. It had real, dark contours and had already shaken two families.

Girls at Jefferson had friends and family members who had been shot or stabbed. Even teachers and administrators weren't immune to violence. I'll never forget a morning when I was counseling freshmen and a distraught student decided to hold Jefferson's principal at gun-point. The principal somehow managed to persuade the student to hand over his gun. Even Erica, just five feet tall and a hundred pounds, sometimes carried a knife to school because she wanted to protect herself. "People are getting killed around here. . . . One of the kids around my house pulled a knife on me," she confided. Her cousin had recently been shot, and the apartment where she lived with her aunt and sister had been robbed several times. Erica found relief from life's dangers by shooting baskets at the outdoor court at Jefferson: "It's good — you don't think about anything when you're playing bas-ketball. I just let it go."

"Stress" is an ever-recurring word in teen language, and not one used lightly. Regardless of economic status or family dynamics, all girls reported feeling considerable stress in their lives. Teens at Jefferson, especially those in my freshman counseling groups, were more likely to mention very tangible and sometimes dramatic pressures. They wor-ried about how their family would make that month's rent, about get-ting beaten up on the way to school, about having enough money to buy clothes. As one girl heartbreakingly put it, "I worry because I don't think there's much hope."

While girls at Nottingham did not face the same level of commu-nity violence as those at Jefferson, girls at both schools feared the po-tential for random disaster to strike their lives. Thirteen-year-old Car-rie described her nightmare that her mom would die while she was still young. Vicki, who first claimed to have no anxieties, later con-ceded, "Well, maybe I'm scared of slow death. I want to die quick." Others worried about their family's stability. Each girl traveled with her own dark cloud of worry, which might have seemed far-fetched to an objective eye but was exceedingly real to her.

The desire to feel safe, loved, and cared for is so basic that girls of-ten do not articulate it as one of their main concerns. When their families cannot fulfill these needs, they may search for other ways to fulfill them. Some young women turn to sexual intimacy, alcohol, il-licit drugs, or tobacco in hopes of alleviating their feelings of loneli-ness.

Despite widespread public health campaigns, tobacco and alcohol continue to be used by a substantial proportion of adolescents and even younger children. In addition, "clusters" of high-risk behaviors, such as tobacco and alcohol use combined with sexual activity, are more prevalent among teens today. In a survey of 750 girls between the ages of twelve and nineteen, for instance, 85 percent identified drinking as a major factor leading to sex. A recent newspaper article entitled "Getting Ready (or Not) for Sex" quoted a seventeen-year-old girl saying, "People use alcohol as an excuse. . . . I was drunk." She elaborated, "If someone wants to [have sex] but doesn't want to face the consequences, they use the alcohol as an excuse. They can't say I consciously made this decision." Almost uniformly, the adolescents in the focus groups reported that their decision to have sex was spontaneous or the result of getting carried away, often aided by alcohol. Ruth had observed a similar phenomenon with her peers: "Getting drunk and having sex sort of go together."[4]

Such words are a wake-up call for us all. Girls are forfeiting their own decision-making processes to the whims of alcohol, and in an odd twist, they feel that drinking allows them to retain some self-respect if they *do* have sex. This intersection of lust and alcohol can be a potent combination, one that even the "best" of girls can be seduced by.

## Knowing the Right Time

If some girls are using alcohol to abdicate responsibility for having sex, many others are just plain confused about how to know the right time to become sexually active. Their confusion teeters between hopeful anticipation and high anxiety. The girls who were not yet sexually active discussed, debated, analyzed, and contemplated endlessly how they would decide on the right time for sexual intercourse and how they would ensure that the moment was satisfying both physically and emotionally. "It looks so perfect in the movies. You don't want it to be a letdown when you finally have sex," one explained.

Though girls wished for candid discussions with their parents on sex, they were not willing to put their most personal decisions in their parents' hands. Even the youngest in the group thought that decisions about relationships should be made independently of their mothers' visions for them. Most reported that if they decided to become sexually active in the near future, they would not speak to their moms about the decision or seek assistance. Even in those cases where moms had made themselves available for discussion, girls didn't want to risk their mothers' disapproving response.

If most of their moms hoped their daughters would abstain from sex in high school and, perhaps, until marriage, the girls thought they would probably wait until near the end of high school but not until marriage. "It depends," said Ingrid. "It may be a good thing to wait until marriage before you're sexually active, but if you don't get married until you're thirty-five years old, that's pretty unrealistic." Not yet prepared to accept the risks of sexual activity, she bargained that her feelings might well change in time: "You fall in love, and your heart and emotions start to overrule your mind."

Ruth was especially adamant that the decision was up to her: "When I become sexually active, it will be *my* decision — me and whomever I am with. It won't be my friends or my mom — no one else except the guy and me, but more myself." To Cindy Gordon's mind, a person "is ready for sex when she thinks she's ready and mature enough to take responsibility and to handle what may occur." Cindy and her friends were aware of the dangers, but they also suspected that at some point near the end of high school or in college they would say yes to sex. "I feel like everybody has done it but me and my cousin," Erica said. "But I'm not sweating it . . . because I want to feel clean inside of me, not nasty."

Fifteen-year-old Katrina found it frustrating to figure out the right time, right age, and right frame of mind for sex: "I wish there was some sort of checklist with some easy answers." When she explored what that list might include, she put a high priority on values, asking, "Does being sexually active at this time in my life fit with my values?" She also noted the importance of having time to develop a caring friendship with her partner and considering whether the relationship would be a long-term commitment. She talked about needing to address with the partner how important it was to use contraception "both ways," where they would find it, and what his previous sexual history had been. The checklist, Katrina thought, also ought to include something about being willing to deal with the potential consequences of sex, including pregnancy and AIDS.[5]

Katrina and some of the older girls were inquisitive about the whole notion of what constituted "normal" for sex and sexuality. They understood there was no one model, that "normal" women expressed their sexuality in different ways, in ways that were right for them. But they wanted some assurance about whether it was "normal" to feel confused about sex and sexuality at this time in their lives.

Many girls want to move slowly in exploring their sexual selves and need help in knowing how to set limits effectively. Sometimes these young women seemed less worried about the consequences of having sex than about the particular conditions under which they might explore sexuality. They wondered, for example, whether boys would like them more or less if they had sex. How would a couple that wanted sex decide to act on their desire? Where would it happen? Were there more gradual steps to take and enjoy with a boyfriend before having sex? What were some of the alternatives? I longed to tell them, Yes, you can take gradual steps to intimacy, that it can exist without that ultimate event. That even kissing can be one of the most intimate things a couple can do.

These perpetual questions aside, they all understood in their own ways that they should expect nothing less than respect from boys. "I want the relationship. I want someone I can feel comfortable with," Kit said with great feeling. In general, the girls were angry at boys who pressured them to have sex or to engage in other activities that made them feel uncomfortable. "If a guy pressures me to do something I don't want to do," Samantha insisted, "I'm just like NO. And if they don't agree with me, I just leave." Erica had dated a boy who told her that he didn't want to go out with her anymore "because he wasn't getting it." She told him, "Fine, I don't need to see you or talk to you anymore."

From what I observed of Anita and Melinda, who were sexually active, both of these young women felt empowered and entitled to engage in a sexual relationship. I never had the sense that they felt pressured by their boyfriends. In fact each of them mentioned that they thought it was foolish for a girl to have intercourse in the early stages of dating a boy because he would be likely to drop her after they had gone all the way.

Tina, on the other hand, seemed quite vulnerable to sexual exploitation. She was so needy and so anxiously searching for love that she was willing to believe almost anyone. As Pauline Dickinson kept reminding her, she was just going to have to put the past behind her and take charge of her life, but that would take some time. Tina believed that the older guy she had begun dating loved her as she loved him, and "someday they were going to get married."

Erica, at fourteen, also was dating someone older — a twenty-one-year-old man who was in college. She had stopped dating boys her own age because "up to about, say, seventeen, they're really immature." Her new boyfriend "treats me like a person and somebody. He doesn't rush the relationship. We talk a lot and we're getting to know about each other's backgrounds," she explained. When Erica told me about this new, thrilling relationship, what came to my mind was the recent research highlighting bad outcomes for teenage girls who date older men. Though not every man who is older will lead a daughter astray, when it comes to teen pregnancies, older males have a strong showing in the father category. In a 1995 survey, researchers found that half of the fathers of babies born to women between fifteen and seventeen were twenty or older. Reinforcing the point, a California survey of 47,000 births to teenage mothers in 1993 determined that 66 percent of the babies were fathered by men of post–high school age. With high school mothers, the fathers tended to be an average of 4.2 years older, and with mothers in junior high school, dads were on average 6.7 years older.[6]

Even though Erica and her boyfriend were taking time to get to know each other, a seven-year age difference can make it difficult for a young adolescent girl to determine her own needs in a relationship. It stands to reason that a fourteen-year-old doesn't possess nearly the experience, skills, or knowledge of someone seven years older. I had an uneasy feeling that beneath the confident exterior and tough talk Erica was a needy girl, and I worried that this man, whom, granted, I didn't know, was preying on her vulnerability.

All the girls who talked about relationships stressed wanting to feel special in them. Several, including Erica, highlighted the difference between "having sex" and "making love." Vicki was sure she wouldn't "fall for any guy who goes, like, 'Come on, come over here and do this or do that.' " In her plucky manner she elaborated: "He would have to be nice to me and have to care for me, and we'd have to have a good relationship. He would have to love me as much as I loved him, and if he insisted I go all the way with him, that wouldn't go with me."

A relationship that creates a seemingly safe and reassuring space for a girl to test out her emerging womanliness understandably becomes precious. It offers companionship, a reaffirmation of her sense of worth, and some of those exciting feelings that Katrina described as "something you'd just like to bottle." While there is a certain thrill in succumbing to the seductions of a take-charge Lothario, the girls were still holding out for control in their romantic encounters. "I like it when a boy says, 'Can I kiss you?' instead of just moving on you," Kit said, "because when they ask, you have control and they do too." Her friends nodded in agreement. "We want to be the ones who get to say what's going to happen. We want to have the control . . . the power to say what's right and wrong."

## Averting Pregnancy and Disease

Every girl I spoke with at Jefferson and Nottingham knew she was supposed to avoid getting pregnant at all costs. When the girls spoke of pregnancy, though, they seemed to fear their parents' reaction more than the pregnancy itself. Vicki, at thirteen, for instance, dreaded the thought of her parents' potential outrage. "I know my mother would kill me. If not my mother, my father. They'd probably have fights over who was going to hit me first." None mentioned pregnancy in any way except as something to avoid, something that would make their parents terribly upset.

Jenny King described the young pregnant girls at her church as wasted potential, and here her words mirrored those of her mother: "I feel so sad for those girls. I mean one girl that had a baby at my church . . . she had this dancing scholarship and she could do so much. She was really a good dancer. But she went off and had two babies by the age of sixteen. It's sad; it's like wasted talent. . . . It's not so bad to have a baby, but it should be reserved for people who are . . . not necessarily married, but people who are adults, because it's an adult action."

Recently we have seen some alarming accounts of teenage girls giving birth and attempting to dispose of their infants without anyone's knowing.[7] The girls' parents deny knowing about the pregnancy. Tragically, some infants have died, and the teen mothers now face trial for homicide. These cases appear to be exceptions. In my work with adolescent girls, I have found that most who get pregnant do tell their mothers, even though they often feel, as one young woman said, "it was one of the hardest things I ever did."

The one worry that upstaged teen pregnancy, however, was AIDS. A few cited "and other diseases," but it was the specter of AIDS that loomed largest. As one girl put it, "Getting pregnant is scary, but getting AIDS is way beyond scary." The girls' strategies for keeping themselves safe from pregnancy, AIDS, and other STDs was not abstinence but information and contraception.[8]

But the girls in the focus groups who were already pregnant indicated that they hadn't quite believed the messages about protecting themselves.[9] It's not that they lacked information, for most were familiar with condoms and other forms of contraception. But it's one thing to know and another thing to obtain contraception and use it correctly. At a workshop I attended on sex and sexuality for professionals who counsel young people about these issues, someone asked, "When's the last time you tried negotiating using a condom and/or birth control with someone?" We know it's a complicated process even with mature adults, and yet we hope that if our adolescent daughters do have sex they will negotiate these very issues. Even if they have the knowledge and can easily obtain contraception, there's still more to the story. Over and over I heard from pregnant teens, "I just didn't think it would happen to me." Sometimes girls seemed to have convinced themselves that mere hope or denial was a form of contraception.

## Facing the World with Exuberance

If we could weigh hopes and fears on a scale, no doubt the scale would tilt toward hope. True, adolescent girls are not carefree souls in a world of sunshine and frolic; fears shadow each one. But Ingrid's exuberance, Angela's drive, Ruth's thoughtfulness, Jenny's enthusiasm, Cindy's spunkiness — this was the armor the girls wore to ward off evil and sustain themselves. Some led extremely difficult lives in dangerous neighborhoods, but what was encouraging was that they continued to care about themselves and about the others in their lives. They had taken up the challenge of adolescence, were in the process of getting an educational foundation, balancing their hopes and fears, figuring out how they felt about their sexuality, and doing their best to survive — and flourish — amid the everday perils. Did their mothers, I wondered, feel the same way?

# SEVEN

# With an Eye Toward Independence

## MOTHERS' HOPES

## AND FEARS

❀

Could it be that we swell large during pregnancy not just with amniotic fluid but with all our hopes and dreams for the baby inside us? Before our children are even out of the womb, we start considering their health and happiness, and once they're in our arms, we plan and plot the joys we hope life will bring them. We watch them grow with wonder and applaud their every accomplishment.

This boundless mother love brimmed over in the conversations I had with women. Mary Robbins spoke of her enormous pride and delight in Vicki's every achievement. When Cybil Mason extolled Bettina's successes, the fierceness of her love was palpable. Alma Parks glowed with affection when she described Angela's leadership roles at Jefferson. That deep, rich, dizzying maternal love was a bond we all shared. We all knew what it meant to love a child so hard it sometimes took away our breath.

As adolescents, they continue to take our breath away — sometimes with their accomplishments, sometimes with their love, sometimes with the outlandish things they do. Suddenly they are dating, driving, and making decisions independently. If we say no, they may, in a moment of despair, scream that they hate us, convincing us that we're unfit parents. Betty Graham had experienced this sudden and surprising animosity with thirteen-year-old Camille; Gerry Valentia felt the sting of Carolyn's words; Diane Early sometimes felt exasperated, as if she could do nothing right when Melinda turned thirteen. Daughters, newly focused on their own concerns, usually can't fathom their mothers' lonely plight as they watch their girls begin the amazing transformation into womanhood.

As each mother shared her aspirations for her daughter, a subtle pattern began to emerge. A mother would begin, full of enthusiasm and animation, to paint a colorful portrait of her daughter's blossoming potential. She would speak first about wanting her girl to enjoy good health, to develop positive self-esteem, to be well educated, and someday have a satisfying career that would provide financial independence. Eventually she would highlight the importance of her daughter's having a caring and loving relationship in which sex was a positive component, and someday a strong family.

In outlining their tremendous hopes, however, some of the moms, especially those who were divorced, began to suggest that they worried about the signals their girls might be picking up from them regarding relationships. Cybil Mason recounted how a child psychologist had told her and her ex-husband that their "child will absorb our relationships and will learn about relationships through us. We sort of swallowed hard and went, 'Whoooah!' But it was a wonderful thing because I realized that every relationship I have is under observation, and they are fertile ground for Bettina and me to discuss relationships."

When the conversations turned to their daughters' current and potential relationships with men, mothers' words took on a darker tone. Not a few used examples from their own pasts to give shape to their worries. Gerry Valentia vividly recalled every ridiculous thing she had done as a teen and imagined, in the same detail, every outrageous thing Carolyn might do. Liana Lee, raised in Taiwan, said her daughter's coming of age called up old tapes she hadn't realized were still playing. "It's been very difficult for me. I come from a country and a culture that has a different set of rules. I grew up with these rules firmly engraved in my mind. It seems they are still there."

## Feeling Good about Herself

Any one of the mothers interviewed might have spoken Joan Rankin's wish for fourteen-year-old Carmen: "I want her to grow up and be happy with who she is and whatever she does in life, whatever she chooses." Or they might have expressed Gerry Valentia's hopes for Carolyn: "I want her to find herself and feel good about herself because if you feel good about yourself, you can do anything you want."

Betsy Gordon, who recalled burying her own selfhood during early adolescence because the adults in her household, especially her mother, didn't approve of assertive girls, applauded and encouraged Cindy's and her sister's feistiness. "I just feel that you can always kind of calm someone down, but you can't give them that spunk. I like that a lot — it's probably because I kept it inside so long myself." Betsy likewise placed a high priority on Cindy's being able "to keep feeling good about herself." "I love her personality," Betsy explained. "She has a good sense of self, and she feels confident about herself. I just hope nothing happens to that."

Gerry Valentia and Betty Graham conveyed similar sentiments about sustaining their daughters' fun-loving natures. They said they sometimes had to bite their tongues to keep from criticizing their girls, particularly when they themselves were the targets of the adolescent jibes.

Many were aware of the battle for teenage girls to maintain a positive sense of themselves in today's society. Whether or not they were familiar with the research, they sensed intuitively what their daughters were up against in adolescence, especially in school. And they recognized that strong self-esteem would help their daughters make good choices in their lives.

The discouraging news is that mothers have their work cut out for them if they are to outshout the cultural messages girls are awash in, the most dominant of which is that you must look beautiful, smell sweet, and smile with perfect teeth if you hope to compete in the game called romance. Susan Harter, a psychologist who has focused a lifetime of research on self-esteem, concludes that whether we are five or fifty-five, the number-one predictor of high self-esteem is our perception of our physical appearance. While girls might have garnered praise for being fast or smart or clever in grade school, as they begin middle school that emphasis shifts to beauty and popularity. As Peggy Orenstein discovered in her examination of eighth-grade girls, intelligence and articulateness were often negatively characterized by the adults in their lives, and as a result these girls were "dumb[ing] themselves down to avoid threatening other girls, boys, and adults." It can be devastating for a bright young teenager who has been cherished by her classmates in grade school not to fit in with the popular crowd in middle school. And this ostracism can be equally devastating for her mother if she follows the aphorism "A mother is only as happy as her most miserable child."[1]

These lessons rang painfully true for me one day when my daughter found a note in her locker, neatly typed and folded. Apparently there was a girls' club at the school that voted on all the new girls in sixth grade. They wanted her to know, the note said, that the club had taken a vote on her — she had gotten zero votes. I was so angry when Katherine told me this that I contemplated an immediate and possibly lethal search for the girl who owned the typewriter with the faulty zero key. But when we want so desperately to protect our daughters, we must also have faith that they will learn to fend for themselves.

## Standing on Her Own Two Feet

Whether they lived in the inner city or in a well-groomed suburb, all mothers, rich and poor, black and white, single or married, shared the conviction that education and financial independence before marriage would help their daughters find happiness. It was clear that their words had helped shape their daughters' thoughts as well. Liana Lee and Alma Parks had drastically different life experiences, but both emphasized that their daughters should become self-sufficient before moving into a serious relationship, marriage, and family. Not one mom, when asked where she envisioned her daughter at twenty-five, imagined that she would be married.

Like their daughters, Marian Henderson, Evelyn Shepherd, and Phyllis Rosenbloom all cited education as the nonnegotiable element in establishing self-sufficiency and economic independence. By the same token, sixty-year-old Pauline Dickinson had not gone past eight grade in school, but when her niece, Tina, expressed an interest in going to college, Pauline told her, "I am going to get it for you."

Mary Robbins, the polished lawyer who was trying to keep up with Vicki's little-girl and early adolescent shifts, likewise counted on Vicki's attending college and graduate school. "I'm not sure what she will choose, but I just feel as a parent, it's up to me to provide her with the kind of windows and opportunities so she can select later." In Alma Parks's home, the importance of an education for her three daughters and her son was hammered home; education would give them a fair shot at getting "decent jobs" and becoming "somebody." In short, these women were teaching their girls not to depend on a man for financial security or emotional well-being. And, as I had heard from the girls, they were absorbing these messages well. There are without a doubt mothers who believe romance is riches and who concentrate their hopes on their daughters' finding a Prince Charming, but weddings were not at the forefront of discussion for the women with whom I spoke.

Looming in the minds of many mothers was the potential that a sexual relationship would derail a girl from her goals. Marian Henderson, for example, did not want Tiffany "thrown off track" by romantic encounters: "Right now she's a very good student and very focused. I worry that something will happen or somebody will come along and distract her and steer her away from what I think is the right course for her." She underscored that she didn't want a young man to diminish Tiffany's sense of her own self-worth. "She is an extremely affectionate person, and I think she could be a child who if someone said, 'I love you,' it would be easy for her to believe that."

In conversation after conversation, mothers recognized how tempting it can be for a young woman to give herself to a boy she loves, who promises to love her — and how much a girl will strive to care for someone who is important to her and make sure that he will always be hers. Estelle Brown, for instance, worried that Sam was too immature even at seventeen to judge the motives of a potential suitor: "If there happened to be a guy that she really liked, and he wasn't *really* a good guy for her, I'm not sure right now what her judgment would be."

With the exception of Alma Parks — who wasn't at all sure that it was a good idea to get permanently entangled with *any* man — mothers fully expected that their daughters would someday marry and have children. They all wanted their girls to have caring, loving relationships and families of their own — but not until the girls had obtained the education they needed.

Emily Shattuck was confident that her gifted daughter would finish college and choose a meaningful career. Yet she also spoke wistfully of wanting something more for Katrina. "I very much want her to be a wife and mother. I think if she didn't marry and have children, I would be extremely disappointed for her because I think that for a woman, that's just . . . everything."

## Pregnancy and AIDS

Mothers' expectant faces began to change as they shifted from their hopes and dreams for their daughters to their sweeping concerns. When they began to reflect on their daughters' relationships with young men, the transformation was unmistakable. Their animation inevitably dimmed, and the worries spilled out, the most central being pregnancy and disease.

For mothers, adolescent pregnancy was still the number-one concern. In one woman's words, "Pregnancy should still be every parent's biggest worry." These mothers knew that teens who get pregnant are less likely to complete their educational goals, less likely to develop financial independence, and less likely to find satisfactory career opportunities. "Because she is mature enough at this point to know about physical attraction and sex, I think our biggest fear is that if she is really attracted to a boy, she might go as far as sexual intercourse. There could be pregnancy and disease." These were the thoughts of Liana

Lee, but they might have been those of any of the mothers interviewed. They agonized over the powerful attraction sex would have for their girls one day, and not a few recalled their younger selves as the basis for their fears. Marian, for instance, had become sexually active at seventeen, but she "lucked out and did not get pregnant."

The mothers' sharp memories of their own adolescent years came flooding back in technicolor when they talked with their daughters about issues of growing up. Liana Lee described how in her adolescence in Taiwan, you "socialized at home, under your parents' eyes." She didn't have her first date until she was twenty-eight, with the man who would eventually become her husband. So when Nicole, at fifteen, wanted to invite a boy home for dinner, Liana was adamantly opposed. "I was surprised with myself that I felt such intense anger about this," she confided. She truly wanted to strike a more balanced approach, but her own upbringing kept intruding.

Just as Marian based her maternal concern on her own early sexual activity, another mother, who had given up a baby for adoption when she was an adolescent, wanted to protect her daughter from a similar debacle. With tears rolling down her face, she described the extraordinarily painful story of how she had known so little and become pregnant. For "a moment of fun," she said, she now had to "suffer the consequences for the rest of her life." She spoke of how she continued to grieve this loss and even now yearned to explain to her lost child why she had gone through with the adoption — and how much love she still felt.

Although pregnancy was the primary worry for moms, they diverged in the ways they conveyed that message to their girls. A few, like Joan Rankin, focused on their daughters' avoiding sexual intimacy altogether until marriage. "No, I will not march my daughter off to a clinic for birth control pills. I wouldn't take her to my doctor," she insisted. "I wouldn't supply her with anything. . . . I don't really want to see her sleeping with somebody before she is married. I think it's wrong." While most of the other mothers preferred that their daughters wait until marriage, many knew that this was probably a pipe dream. Marian Henderson conceded, "That's not, I feel, realistic in today's world. I would ask if at all possible that she not have sex in high school because I don't think that a sixteen- or seventeen-year-old is ready for that."

As uncomfortable as some mothers were in explicitly advocating the use of contraceptives, in general they had come to terms with this issue. They felt it would be much worse if their daughters became sexually active and did not protect themselves. "No siree," one mother told her daughter, "we don't need any more mouths to feed in this house." She favored straight talk: if her daughter wanted to go to a clinic to get birth control, she should just say the word.

For many mothers, especially those in single-parent households, the economic, as well as the emotional, costs of pregnancy were pre-eminent. Some talked frankly with their girls about what would happen after the baby was born. Who would care for it? How would their daughters manage financially? Gerry Valentia didn't mince words: "I'm pushing fifty," she warned her girls, "and I am not ready to deal with a child so don't bring me home a baby. I don't think it's fair of you to expect me to raise it, and neither do I want to see you out there struggling — because it would break my heart."

Nor did Julie King hesitate to make her expectations crystal clear to Jenny. "I have told her that it's tragic, *very tragic*, that a young girl who has not experienced anything of life and knows very little, finds she is pregnant and about to be a mother," explained Julie. "I say to her, 'I hope and pray that you will never experience this and you're aware this is not what you want for your life.'" Jenny had described teen pregnancy earlier to me in much the same way.

While parents across generations have understood the threat of pregnancy, it is the scourge of AIDS, as we saw earlier, that has dramatically shifted conversations about sex. Pauline Dickinson had never worried about AIDS when her own daughter was growing up, but after becoming Tina's legal guardian she was confronted by a much more frightening and complicated world for adolescents. "Somebody needs to do something," she insisted, "because nowadays the kids are too sexually inclined. . . . You don't know if these fellows you're going out with have AIDS or not. You could die." Marian Henderson declared, "I am very scared about the AIDS epidemic. I don't want Tiffany to feel as though sex is not a pleasurable experience, but I don't want her to think of it as recreation either." For some the danger of AIDS was what had compelled them to talk with their daughters about sex in the first place. Mothers believed they no longer had a choice but to take up the subject. All had talked with their daughters about AIDS, often using school materials to initiate discussion.

## Manipulated and Exploited

Mothers may be distressed for daughters who lack the qualities that lead to teen acceptance and popularity, but on the flip side, what are they to do when a daughter seems to beguile others too easily? Gerry Valentia was thrilled to see Carolyn's success after her years of struggling, but by the same token she worried that Carolyn's new self-confidence could be a disadvantage: "The only fear I have is that she will talk to anybody — she is so outgoing that it doesn't matter who you are, where you come from, what your status in life is, whether you're a criminal or a saint — Carolyn will talk to you."

Dorothy Dodson, a divorced mother, shared similar anxieties about Anita, who was involved in a stable relationship with a young man. "She's really affectionate with people, and sometimes that scares me. I always worry that she could be suckered in so easily." Many mothers thought their daughters somewhat naive and overly trusting. Mary Robbins, for example, considered Vicki's nonjudgmental nature to be a plus, but her words paralleled another mother's: "She could get hurt by someone who takes advantage or manipulates her — an emotional injury would be very hard for her."

Most agreed that their daughters were not yet mature enough to exercise sound judgment in their relationships with boys. And thus most of them discouraged their daughters from dating anyone on a regular basis at this time. The Nottingham girls' busy schedules conveniently enhanced their mothers' wishes. With extracurricular activities oftentimes running until 6:30 and into weekends, they had little time for dating. At Jefferson, however, the school day ended at 1:30 for most students, with fewer extracurricular activities available. A few of the girls had part-time jobs, but they seemed to have plenty of time to hang out with their girlfriends and boys.

One mother described how her fourteen-year-old daughter had begun seeing a boy on a very regular basis, and she thought some very passionate feelings were beginning to be tapped: "Things had gotten hot and heavy," she said. When the boyfriend came over to their house to do homework, she insisted that her daughter's bedroom door stay open.

Despite their mothers' fears, to be fair, the daughters thought their moms underestimated their ability to make good decisions and maintain control in a dating situation. Almost all were as adamant as their moms about the importance of staying in control when they were on a date.

Mothers expressed particular concern, however, if their daughters were seeing young men who were significantly older, and they were quick to let their girls know their views. When Sam, at sixteen, started dating a man whom Estelle thought was in his early twenties (he told Sam he was nineteen), Estelle, usually quiet on such matters, said her piece. "We bumped heads over this one. She knew I strongly disapproved so she pulled back. She never agreed with me," Estelle explained. "But I thought that his experience and his maturity and his ability to do things that she was not experienced with, and hopefully not ready for . . . I could see many things happening." Estelle was greatly relieved when Sam eventually did stop seeing him. Boys one or two years older than their daughters were not such a worry; young men four to six years older gave mothers great pause. Their instincts told them that their daughters shouldn't get involved.

Mothers may take comfort in learning that some states have taken steps to increase the prosecutions of adults who have sexual intercourse with underage youth even when it is consensual. For example, under Pennsylvania's statutory rape law, anyone who has sexual intercourse with a person under thirteen is guilty of rape, a first-degree felony. The law also provides that anyone who has sexual intercourse with an adolescent under sixteen and who is four or more years older than the sexual partner (and not married to her or him) is guilty of statutory sexual assault, a felony of the second degree.[2]

The clear legal restraints that have been enforced of late in many states allow parents and other adults, in a quiet and private way, to explain to any older male who is dating a younger girl that having sexual intercourse is not only against the law but subject to severe criminal punishment. To protect young girls against sexual manipulation, recent legislative hearings have encouraged better sex education in schools and broader community support.[3]

Mothers also fretted that their daughters might become victims of violence. The Jefferson moms, in particular, worried that their daughters were at risk for being raped, shot, stabbed, or killed. And for some, it was a very personal fear; the mother of a Jefferson girl said she had been raped when she was an adolescent, and the mother of a Nottingham student had been attacked when she had gone out on a date with someone she thought she knew well. Neither had yet shared her experience with her daughter. "It's the kind of thing that just seems like too much," one mother painfully explained. They wanted their girls to be aware of the potential for sexual abuse, but they didn't want to unduly scare them. One mother in the group had signed herself and her daughter up for a self-defense course.

Even when girls date their peers and are in relatively "safe" relationships, mothers worry about the pain and disillusionment their daughters may experience if they are "dumped" by the boy. Evelyn Shepherd cautioned Ingrid about the likelihood of heartbreak if she were to become sexually involved with a boy who left her for someone else. Mothers knew intuitively that girls are usually more emotionally bound up in their relationships than boys. They didn't want to see their young daughters at risk for rejection.

But it may be that the very relationships we fear in fact help girls define themselves and become stronger and more independent. Every girl reacts differently to rejection, disappointment, and deceit. Some teens feel truly heartbroken; others are able to integrate the disappointment and keep moving ahead. Still others bravely challenge perceived disloyalties on the part of their boyfriends. Katrina offered a case in point. There was an "incredible" flirt in her school who couldn't seem to resist her boyfriend. "I'd be like walking down the hall and just right in front of me, she'd start flirting. I told her off 'cause it really annoyed me. Then my boyfriend came up to me and said, 'What did you say to her?'" Their relationship had been put in question by her telling the flirtatious girl how she felt. "I've done my best to put a stop to it, but there's only so much I can do, and it's only my business to a certain extent," she acknowledged.

## The Wrong Crowd

When mothers discussed some of their fears, the phrase "getting in with the wrong crowd" emerged often. As teens try to shape their adolescent identity, peer groups can provide invaluable support systems and the coveted stamp that they are "okay." But as Betty Graham also understood, girls will sometimes tolerate behavior they know is inappropriate or agree to activities that make them uncomfortable because they fear rejection by their friends. She worried that Camille's desire to become a member of the "cool" group would lead her to keep company with teens who were smoking, drinking, and engaging in other dangerous activities. Some parents made a point of cautioning their girls directly, such as Betsy and Stan Gordon, who warned Cindy and her sister about drug and alcohol abuse. Many saw these behaviors as directly connected to their daughters' friends.

## Getting to a Good Place

Adolescent girls today are coming of age in an era of rapidly expanding opportunities for females. Women on the Supreme Court, in the military, or on a national-league basketball team, all images perfectly familiar to our daughters, were unfathomable when many of us were born. So much change in a relatively short period of time makes it difficult to know which of our hopes and fears are reasonable and which are not.

The choices open to women have altered drastically, and so have our expectations for girls. As one successful executive, wife, and mother sadly confided, "My mother devoted herself to cleaning the house, raising the children, and caring for my father — she was good at it. But for some reason she sees my life as a working wife and mother as a negation of what she did. And, instead of being proud of me, she seems to look for ways to put me down."

Mothers like Alma Parks saw in their daughters young women who would build interesting careers, become financially independent, and take charge of their lives. Knowing that the choices daughters make in their teen years will have long-term effects, mothers naturally worry, especially about the bad consequences. What they can take heart in, however, is that adolescence is a learning curve for all involved and that much of what they say to their daughters is coming through loud and clear.

# EIGHT

# Speaking
# the Unspoken

## SEXUAL DESIRE

**D**esire. Just the word conjures up images of moonlight trysts, romantic getaways, and passionate yearnings for things within our reach — and beyond it. Desire drives us, inspires us, and sometimes haunts us. If passion is so close to us, then why, when we women try to discuss desire among ourselves, do we often become tongue-tied or oddly silent? If it is a normal aspect of our lives, shouldn't it be a part of our conversations? It sounds logical, but for most women, giving voice to desire in our everyday lives is akin to revealing our most intimate secrets. Even those of us who enjoy steamy romance novels and seductive movies are silent about the desirous passions in our own minds or personal relationships.

How can adult women learn to speak easily of desire with their closest female friends? Some surely do, but for most it is exceedingly difficult. One woman who participated regularly in a women's discussion group noted that "while the group spent many meetings talking about their bodies and their particularities, the erotic contours of our imaginations remained buried in layers of propriety and ambivalence. Face to face when it came to describing our desires, we were strangely mute."[1] If we do speak, our words tend to dissipate the passion and the particulars. That's not to say locker-room talk is the wave of women's liberation around desire — but it would be nice to have a certain comfort zone. Even when I spoke with another mother on how to address desire with a daughter the two of us — grown women — would giggle, lower our eyes, and blush at the suggestion of such an intimate and personal subject.

We live in a society in which female sexual desire still carries with it the ominous luster of something slightly taboo and off-limits. As Naomi Wolf in her book *Promiscuities* and the authors of *Mother-Daughter Revolution* point out, our culture is quick to label young women as either "good girls" or "bad girls." Teens quickly become either the sexually innocent and desire-free or, alternatively, the sexually active and desire-ridden. If we think about the odd mathematics this suggests, more than half of the girls in this country are "bad" by the time they emerge from their teens.[2] We know these labels register powerfully with girls like Ruth, who thought hinting at her own sexual desire would make her mother think she was not "a good person."

An unusual public comment in a college alumnae bulletin further drives the point home. Two adult women who now work with teens described their own experiences in adolescence: "Both of us had been dating our partners for at least a year before we began, carefully, to consider whether to have sex; both [of us] sought family planning services before losing our virginity and both stayed happily in these relationships for several years." The authors recalled their high school experiences as "some of our most sexually rewarding" but wrote that "society makes us feel uncomfortable about the satisfaction and pleasure we experienced as young women. . . . Conventional wisdom tells us our relationships were unusual, although many other women we know share our experience."[3]

In recent years we have made some headway in acknowledging that girls may *feel* desire, but they had better not talk about it and most certainly had better not act on it — or they will be tagged as "bad girls." But we continue to perpetuate a negative label if we use a term like "bad girl" in order to fully participate in desire. The expectation that women are either "bad" or "good," loose or chaste, confuses the issue and leads us into troubling semantics. Why is it that desire cannot be a natural part of a woman's life? Isn't being desirous an element of being a woman just as much as it is part of being a man? That men have desire is an assumption that has been accepted with little argu-ment for centuries. Women today can actively resist categorization into the "good" or "bad" slot; it is time for us to recognize and let others know that we are all real girls and real women who experience desire as a wonderful and empowering part of our human makeup.

The question remains, how can we help our daughters recognize and embrace their sexual desire without leading them to sex? Many of us know from our own adolescent relationships the seductiveness of sex. Gerry Valentia spoke of having "given in" as a young woman and later concluding that "it wasn't worth it." She thought it best to steer her girls away from sexual intimacy in adolescence, since she knew how easily passion can push aside rationality and responsibility: "You look into his eyes and BINGO, the sirens go off, and you can't turn back. . . . I don't think it matters at the time if you have contraception or you don't or even if the person might have AIDS. . . . You're turned on, you're ready to go, and you're not thinking."

Traditionally, American society has deigned female desire accept-able so long as it is considered in the context of reproduction. The do-main of motherhood takes away the sexiness of female desire. It has always been "safe" to address issues related to female reproduction — a woman's natural rite. Of all the topics we touched on, the mothers I spoke with had by far the easiest time talking with their girls about re-productive issues. They spoke frankly, abandoning the euphemisms they had learned growing up. Vagina, penis, intercourse, ovulation, ejaculation — words like these were no longer taboo. Girls like Angela Parks, in fact, made a point of using anatomically correct terms. "We have breasts, not titties," Angela said. "And I don't like slang terms. They're rude. I have a nephew and I am teaching him straight to the point, so when he gets a little older, he'll know he has a penis and his Aunt Angela has a vagina."

The fact that we can speak frankly, using the correct terms, on ba-sic reproductive issues signals some strides in mothers' dialogues with daughters. But even this generation of mothers appears unable to use forthright language for the pleasurable aspects of sex. Dalma Heyn wrote of this mysterious quiet in her book *The Erotic Silence of the*

*American Wife*: "Mothers will talk about the mechanics of sex and about the results of careless sex . . . but girls learn no names for their sexual organs."[4] In Heyn's study a favorite euphemism for the female genitalia was "down there." But if we don't name the vagina, then it becomes all the more difficult to name the clitoris, and if we avoid pinpointing the clitoris, we are likely to slide away from addressing female desire and satisfaction altogether.

## Naming Desire

We are confronted by a dilemma in this decade: no one wants to take up the torch to talk about desire with our girls. Mother after mother confessed to me she was stymied about discussing this deepest feeling. Both mothers and daughters reported that the more pleasurable aspects of sex came up seldom, if at all, and were not easy to discuss. Arousal, desire, orgasm, and oral sex were topics on which there was little, if any, communication. A subject "too intimate . . . too inexplicable . . . too private," desire was captured in euphemisms when mothers did broach it with their daughters. Most often, it was something to be wary of: "Don't lose your head in the heat of the moment"; "Keep your head above water"; "Watch your p's and q's"; "Don't cross the line" were common refrains, while "doin' it" was the most popular way to mention intercourse. As Gerry Valentia explained, "We don't use names, but we know what we're talking about."

The assumption that daughters understand what we are speaking of can be dangerous, however. Girls often understand the general direction of their mothers' thinking, but inexact wording can leave the wrong impression. Even with the basics, general phrasing can be problematic. Girls may know they are supposed to "be prepared" for their first sexual encounter, but they may be less sure of what that preparation entails. When it comes to desire, our messages can be all the more confusing.

Mothers believed that by avoiding language that paid tribute to girls' — and perhaps their own — feelings of desire or sexual curiosity they would dissuade their girls from acting on those feelings. Mary

Robbins's mother had told Mary, among other things, that all men are homely, ugly creatures. And when Vicki discovered an old suitcase belonging to one of Mary's aunts with pictures that showed a woman performing fellatio, both Mary and Vicki reported in their interviews that the pictures were "dirty . . . really dirty." Rather than using the photos to discuss the distastefulness of making private intimacies public pornography, Mary, in the spirit of her own mother, apparently felt Vicki would be best served by negative words intended to discourage curiosity.

Even those moms who worked diligently to educate their daughters on reproduction and the risks of pregnancy were embarrassed to speak of desire and the potential pleasures of sex. When Cindy turned fourteen, Betsy Gordon was suddenly uncertain how to direct her conversations about sex. She wanted Cindy to know that "you can have these overpowering emotions and that's wonderful. I don't want her ever to think that's bad because it's not." But Betsy had never discussed any of the pleasure of sex with Cindy. "Orgasm would be something very difficult to talk about because . . . it's so experiential. I knew technically what it was, but the first time it ever happened to me, it was like, Oh, my God! THIS IS IT! . . . I can remember thinking, so this is what everybody was talking about. And it was just totally out of my control. . . . To describe something like that doesn't come anywhere close."

Mothers were afraid of misleading their daughters. Dorothy Dodson, of whom Anita had said "we talk about everything," admitted, "I don't feel comfortable talking to my kids about that. In fact, that was one of the things that was hard. I don't know, I don't think I could. Come on, that's private, you know what I mean? I can't express my feelings on that. I don't think that's fair to them because their expectation of what might happen might be, you know, wrong." She pointed out that on a good day she could joke about it. "I'm shy toward that, but if I was joking, I can joke about it. Like I might say, 'Oh, God, man, I would like to be with this guy tonight. Oh, man he makes me feel good.' . . . But I won't say sexually. . . . I'd just say, 'Oooh, he makes me feel good.' That's about the extent of that."

Betsy, like other mothers, worried that revealing too much about sexual pleasure would lead her daughters to become sexually active. She thought her girls might say, " 'Wow, I've got to try this.' . . . My kids are like that." She elaborated, "If someone says, 'Let's go sky-diving,' they say, 'Great. What time?' This spunkiness makes me nervous when it comes to the sexuality issue." Her daughters, Betsy suspected, would also feel uncomfortable and embarrassed if she tried to have a discussion about sexual pleasures with them.

Marian Henderson, who thought she could talk about most anything with Tiffany, said she would be able to cover orgasm but oral sex would be tougher. "I honestly can't think of anything I wouldn't discuss — not to say that everything has come up. I would like to tell her, 'If you're going to have sex, I want you to have an orgasm.' " After further reflection, she added that some topics could be tough to bring up with a fifteen-year-old: "I might have some reservations about discussing [in a whisper] *oral sex*. . . . I have a very open attitude about sex. I do, but I'm not so sure I want her attitude to be quite so open at such a young age. . . . I don't want to lie to her and tell her I feel one way about something when I don't."

In her own life, Marian took unabashed pleasure in physical intimacy. "I enjoy sex. I expect to enjoy it and feel it is my right to enjoy it. And I want to be sexually active for a very long time. It is one of the pleasures of adult life I would not like to do without." It had taken her many years to arrive at this point, though, and she wanted Tiffany to avoid the shame, hesitancy, and insecurity she had had to sort through. Pleasure had to be balanced with care, caution, and maturity.

Some mothers recognized that discovering desire was a natural part of growing up, and most alluded to the day when their daughters would be able to explore and enjoy their sexuality. Even if they wished to guard their girls from an experience that they felt adolescents weren't emotionally or intellectually prepared for, most hoped that, in Mary Robbins's words, their girls would one day "think sex is a good item." And unlike most of their own mothers, these women were searching for appropriate ways to convey the positive side of sex to their girls, if only in abstract language. Some wanted to make sure that their girls would understand that feelings of arousal and desire are natural and that desire can exist and be expressed without sex. Others emphasized to their daughters that fun and pleasure can accompany sex with someone who cares for you. Mothers were striving to strike a balance by acknowledging that sex can be great but stating that it can also be dangerous and can derail a young girl from her goals.

## The Double Standard of Desire

Why is female eroticism supposed not to exist outside of love and marriage when girls are bombarded by erotic encouragement in the media? There is a double standard at work here.

The girls I interviewed were more quick to justify boys' sexual longings than their own. Ruth, for example, said that she thought girls were really curious about sexual activity, but "it's not that we have to do that, like your hormones are driving you to do this. But with guys, it's like I have to, *now*. And to feel more manly about themselves, they think they've got to have sex before they go to college." She continued, "I talk with my friends and I don't know anyone who feels like the guys do, like I *have* to do this. Like we might say, 'This feels nice,' or 'I like that.' But no one ever says I got really turned on so we had to have sex. I've never heard a girl say that."

Some psychologists, such as Deborah Tolman, contend that our culture teaches girls that they are valued for their sexual desirability and that this lesson makes them particularly vulnerable to the longings and sexual impulses of boys. This vulnerability is compounded by the license given to adolescent boys regarding the urgency of their sexual desire. Just as the culture teaches girls that their desire makes them vulnerable, its message for boys is that their sexuality is too strong to control. This, then, leaves the already vulnerable adolescent girl with the full responsibility for making sexual choices for both herself and her partner. If she fails to regulate her own sexual behavior and her partner's, she becomes a "bad girl." As Tolman points out, "Cultural stories lead girls toward action to satisfying the boy's desire rather than her own. To want anything is to consent to everything."[5]

Circumspection around desire begins at an early age for our daughters. When psychologist Michelle Fine examined the curriculums in New York City sex education classes, she discovered that "a discourse of desire remains a whisper inside the official work of public school. . . . The naming of desire, pleasure, or sexual entitlement, particularly for females, barely exists in the formal agenda of public schooling on sexuality." On the other hand, no one seems to regard masculine urges as too private or personal to discuss. Schools touch on male desire when they include wet dreams, erection, and ejaculation in biology or sex education classes. So it is not that desire is completely unarticulated; it is only *female* desire that gets overlooked. On the rare occasions when it is mentioned, "it is tagged with reminders of 'consequences' — emotional, physical, moral, reproductive and/or financial" for our girls.[6]

Fine's research raises an important question: "If boys learn about erection and ejaculation, how is it then that girls can't learn about the connection between their hormonal cycles and sexual peaks for women? In addition to teaching girls about how the menstrual cycle works and how the cycle is related to the risk of getting pregnant, why not teach them also about how their cycle is related to the sexual drives and urges they experience each month?"[7] Our failure to discuss female sexual desire further disempowers our girls. It takes no stretch of the imagination to understand how a young woman who feels desire but whose feelings are not legitimized or discussed either at home or in school may feel cautious, and perhaps ashamed, about her own natural longings.

Compounding the silence and negative stereotypes surrounding female desire is the meager vocabulary we possess to explain a woman's feelings in all their complexity and richness. In recent years a number of women researchers have noted the negative implications and paucity of words associated with female sexual desire.[8]

Boys, however, seem to be armed with an arsenal of sexual terms at an early age. In a recent comparison of slang terms or euphemisms for male and female desire, girls once again came up short. A query on the Internet about terms used for male and female masturbation produced a list of 457 words and phrases to describe male masturbation and, in stark contrast, only 20 terms for female masturbation. Beyond the disparity in the images, there was also a striking difference in the descriptions of male and female masturbation. The terms used to describe female masturbation often favored traditional womanly characteristics. Many drew upon cooking analogies, such as "making soup," "rolling the dough," and "flicking the bean." Others were more intimate phrases of body pampering: "brushing the beaver," "tickling the taco," or "paddling the pink canoe." Other quirkily nautical descriptions were "making waves for the man in the boat" and "parting the Red Sea." Musical and dance references included "playing the silent trombone," "strumming the banjo," or "doing the two-finger rumba."

In a marked departure from these softer descriptions, terms for boys' masturbation related to more physical, and often more violent, visual images. For example, "bashing" and "beating" were common: "bashing the candle," "beating the stick," "beating your meat." "Choking" was another frequently used verb, as in "choking the chicken" or "choking the sheriff." From "flogging the dong," "flogging the salami," "jerking off," "jerkin' the gherkin" to "whacking the weasel" and "whacking the one-eyed worm," phrases for male pleasure were active and rough. Many of these phrases are probably familiar to our ears, but when juxtaposed with the list for female masturbation, the themes of active battle become all the more apparent.

War images also emerged with regularity: "doing hand battle with the purple-helmeted warrior of love," "holding the sausage hostage," "the one-gun salute." "playing tag with the pink torpedo," and "shining the port sword." Nicknames for condoms similarly carried warrior connotations: missile silo, crash helmet, cloak for dagger, scabbard, bullet bag, and bullet casing. Boys were the undisputed winners for possessing a variety of term for their penises, including such familiar pet names as "peter" and "dick," as opposed to the dearth of terms used by girls for their vaginas.

On a small scale, these lists not only suggest the vast repertoire of terms that boys have developed for sex but also imply the different ways in which boys and girls are thinking about their sexual desire.

What does it say to us when a random survey reveals more than twenty times the number of terms for male masturbation as for female masturbation?[9]

## Saying What We Think

What mothers are willing to say to their daughters about desire — and how they say it — is often influenced by how they regard desire in their own past experiences. Beyond the mother-daughter pairs, I also conducted a small supplemental study of sixty mothers, each of whom had at least one adolescent daughter, to examine mothers' sexual attitudes in greater depth. Of these sixty women, 70 percent were white, 25 percent African American, and 3 percent Hispanic; 70 percent were married, and almost 30 percent were divorced or separated.[10]

These mothers confirmed that sexual activity often began in the teenage years. More than half had engaged in intercourse by the time they left their teens, with the average age of first intercourse around seventeen. Ten had become sexually active at twenty-one, and by the time they were twenty-two, only six of these women had not experienced intercourse.[11]

These mothers looked back on their own adolescent sexual experiences — or lack thereof — with mixed reactions. Roughly a third thought that their adolescent experiences had helped them in their adult relationships, while a quarter believed they had been detrimental. Those who spoke with pleasure of their first sexual encounters highlighted the importance of a loving partner: "My first partner was gentle and loving — it was a positive experience," said one. Another commented, "I had none of the negative emotions associated with teen sexual intercourse."

Those who expressed regret about their adolescent sexual behavior pointed out that it had gotten in the way of other teenage pursuits. "Inappropriate choices interfered with personal growth opportunities," described one. Some voiced regret at not having had sex sooner: abstinence "formed a habit of management and control which led to explo-

ration somewhat late" and "inappropriately." Others confessed that
they had married too young, probably in order to have sex: "I waited
until my wedding night but wish that I hadn't." Another said, "I was
very confused about sex as a teenager. I married quite young and
learned much more about sex with my husband. The first time I really
enjoyed it [sex] was after I had been married several years."

In general, these women gauged whether their sexual initiation
was a positive or negative experience not so much on its timing but on
the quality of the relationship in which it occurred. Whether with a
boyfriend during adolescence or with a husband in their twenties, they
valued being loved, treated with care and respect, and being a full
partner in the decision to become sexually active. Any harmful effects
appeared less closely associated with their age at sexual initiation than
with whether or not they had engaged in behaviors that weren't right
for them.

When it came to their own sexual desire, however, these mothers
seemed more willing to put aside the relationship component. The
majority of responses to the question "What do the words 'sexual desire' first call to your mind?" focused on adjectives of self-gratification,
while a smaller percentage highlighted the importance of intimacy and
love in the context of a strong relationship. Those mothers who responded in terms of self-gratification used such phrases as "having
strong feelings, lust, craving, pleasure and stimulation, attraction, excitement, joy, fun, letting go, and intensity." Some described sexual
desire strictly in terms of wanting to have intercourse: they wanted to
touch and be touched and caressed, to make love with someone who
attracted or aroused them. Those who spoke of sexual desire in the
context of a relationship used expressions such as "the feeling to want
to be intimate with the one I love" or "being crazy in love."

In reviewing their current sex lives, the majority of these women
— nearly 75 percent — viewed it positively and were satisfied with
their partners. Yet 40 percent of them wanted more sex than they currently had; only two of the sixty women indicated that they would like
less sex. About 20 percent considered sex to be "highly overrated" or

said it had become perfunctory in their lives. These women were simply too tired or felt that sex had begun to feel "like grocery shopping" — a routine event.

For some women today sexual desire is still a mystery. A handful of these mothers suggested that they were more or less neutral to the whole idea. One said that sexual desire meant "nothing" to her: "If sex pops into my mind, it pops out." Though she wistfully went on, "At this point in my life I would like for someone to romance me." Another acknowledged feelings of ambivalence: "From a physiological standpoint, I don't know if I've ever had sexual desire. For me it is something that is totally emotional and there is not a physical component to it." Still another mother wrote, "I have never felt that sex was vital to my well-being, but a nice addition. I suspect that I'm pretty normal in my feelings and attitudes."

Importantly, not one expressed feeling "bad" about herself for having feelings of sexual desire or equated sexual desire with anything that could be construed as negative. Yet for many, desire continued to be wrapped up in how men saw them rather than how they envisioned themselves. "My early sexuality was shaped by how boys/men responded to and treated me," wrote one. "My understanding of sex was that it stemmed not from my own desire, but from being desired. I learned objectification."

Another woman alluded to the importance of breaking open the silence on this traditionally private subject: "It took me a long time to understand the concept of love and desire for a man and to give it back because I felt it, too. I am still confused and insecure about certain aspects of myself because so much of myself was not based on organic desire but on the manufactured desire that came from being 'desired' physically — but not loved. I still have trouble recognizing love and real desire. I can still fall into the pattern of defining myself based on how men perceive or respond to me."

Such words carry import for mothers teaching their daughters today. In *Mother-Daughter Revolution*, the authors urge mothers to think back to their own sexual experiences, to remember what they were told about their bodies and how it felt, to recall their experiences, and to take pride in their daughters' desire. "Desire isn't just about sex," they write. "Desire, so often exhausting to adults, holds the force of a girl's embodied self-love — *I want, I need, I love* . . . The greater a girl's connection to the 'yes!' " within herself, the greater a girl's ability to be autonomous, that is, to care for herself." Desire is our girls' to possess. Being desirous begins with the self, and the sooner we can help our girls understand that, the better off they will be in guarding themselves from self-definition through men's eyes.[12]

But how did these women, the overwhelming majority of them reporting positive sexual experiences and a comfort with their own feelings of desire, speak to their adolescent girls about sexual pleasures? How did they differ on this matter from mothers like Gerry Valentia and Betty Graham? The consensus was that it was important to discuss desire, in its broadest sense, with girls. Nearly 40 percent of these mothers responded that girls ought to know about sexual gratification. Yet it was odd: despite all their well-meaning goals to discuss desire, when it came to delivering the message, words were watered down. While one mother responded that she would "absolutely" discuss orgasm with her daughter, most of these mothers mirrored the sentiments of Jefferson and Nottingham mothers on the difficulty of addressing this subject with teen girls. "I wish I could. I think I should," said one mother. "I am the prototype liberated female and can't do this."

Those who advocated talking about it conceded that getting to the specifics was a challenge: "I think it's good to talk about desires . . . when you realize that your daughter begins to have a desire for a boyfriend, but outcomes like orgasm can probably wait until they ask," said one mother. Desire was a safe topic, but orgasms were for later and "better left to college roommates." Another mother found it easier to speak of "sexual excitement" than orgasms.

Some girls have questions about desire at a very early age. One mother reported an intimate conversation with her four-year-old daughter, who "started asking me questions about the penis, such as 'How does it feel going in?' " Another mother was made acutely aware that arousal begins very early when she was driving her preschool daughter to nursery school one morning. "We were driving on this cobblestone street, and as the car bounced along, my daughter called out from the back seat, 'Oh, Mommy, we're on that street that makes my vagina tickle!' "

Some mothers found it easier to have a rapport with older adolescent daughters about sexual issues. One mom told of coming home one evening to find her daughters, in their late teens, watching a movie with a couple of their girlfriends. "The movie was definitely X-rated," she explained. After watching some of it with her daughters and their friends, she ended up having an open conversation with these young women about "the G-spot." Reflecting on this conversation, she noted, "I don't know if it's good or bad, but they're sexually active — that's where we are now."

Her words ring true for many of us. It is difficult to judge whether or not it's right to acknowledge our girls' questions about G-spots. When a nineteen-year-old daughter raises the question, a mother can feel downright ambivalent about how to respond. Although I heard over and over again from mothers how uneasy and uncertain they felt in handling these questions, those who made an effort to respond openly noted some positive results, such as a more open relationship with a daughter or the feeling that they had given a strong signal that they were always available to discuss other topics. A mother may have to take a deep breath and feel her face turn red when speaking of desire, but it is important to have these conversations.

Of course, best intentions don't always bring the results we want. One mother described how she had taken the initiative, but her nineteen-year-old daughter had said no thanks: "I have tried to discuss this with [her] and she says, 'That's okay, Mom, I already know about that stuff. Besides it embarrasses me for you to talk about that kind of stuff. Moms aren't supposed to talk to you about that kind of stuff. You talk with friends about that." Another recounted that she knew she should try to address sexual desire but could never find the time "when my daughter would be comfortable." A few thought their daughters believed raising the issue was "intrusive." Still another echoed Dorothy Dodson's opinion that the mystery of sex is hard to sum up quickly: "I do not believe the desired outcomes should be discussed. It should be left up to the individual to discover."

One thing was clear, however; when mothers do address sexual pleasure, they usually place it in the context of a meaningful relationship. As one mom said, "I don't think physical mechanics should be separated from values regarding intimacy and relationships in general."

Overall, mothers from the supplemental study seemed slightly more comfortable in discussing sexual desire with their girls than those from Nottingham and Jefferson. In part the reason may be that their daughters were slightly older — on average just under sixteen years — than those in my mother-daughter pairs. For older teens these conversations are more urgent, and as girls begin to come back to their mothers after midadolescence, the conversations may become less awkward. Yet these moms suspected, too, that despite their best intentions to make sexual desire "a natural topic to talk about," their daughters detected some of their own confusion and hesitancy.

## Finding Our Own Way

The preventive for premature sexual activity is not silence or avoidance but helping girls understand everything tied up in sex. This means not just the factual information on risks surrounding pregnancy, AIDS, other STDs, and contraception, but what is happening within themselves. When mothers simply caution against "doin' it" or "giving in," they fail to legitimize the good part, the juicy, life-giving component, of these sexual feelings. As these mothers' stories display, we seldom level with them or talk in a meaningful way that will dissipate confusion and frustration. Perhaps what we need is a new vocabulary, of positive and affirming words that can express desire not yet completed, to help our daughters make sense of their feelings.

We could use words similar to those voiced by mothers — "lusting," "longing," "arousal," "excitement" — without assuming that sexual intercourse is the only option for acting on desire. In the same vein, why not employ words like "self-gratification" and "self-touching" in addition to "masturbation" when explaining that it is normal and common for us to touch all of our body parts? We can explain that desire can also be felt and expressed with a partner in intimate gestures of kissing or touching — without going all the way to intercourse.[13] We can reiterate to our girls that embracing sexuality does not necessarily mean having sex.

What might we say to create a positive image for ripe sexuality bound by intelligent restraint? "Virginity" is not a word that legitimizes the duality of desire and restraint, any more than "slut" is appropriate for a girl who simply acknowledges her desire. Intelligent, real women encompass both desire and restraint. We should be able to find the words to express this without resorting to the old bad girl/good girl dichotomy.

If moving away from describing menstruation as a curse has led mothers to celebrate their daughters' entry into womanhood, there should be great potential for finding more positive ways to describe other aspects of a young girl's emerging womanliness. If we begin to listen to the voices of mothers and girls and allow ourselves to discuss sexuality and sexual desire as an important — and given — part of a woman's life and not something to be ashamed of, we will begin to find our way to talking more easily, confidently, and honestly.

Whether or not mothers define and describe orgasm to their mid- or late-adolescent daughters is only one aspect of the issue at hand. Determining the exact stages in a daughter's development to seize opportunities for discussion is a guessing game, but maternal instincts can serve us well here. Certainly, if a four-year-old begins talking about cobblestone streets tickling her vagina, a mother can segue into teaching about arousal and desire. There are some moments to interject thoughts about desire in the preschool and school-age years, but the time to initiate more extensive conversations about desire is right after menarche or when a daughter begins to show interest in dating and curiosity about sexual activity.

Before these conversations, we need to ask ourselves what our own sexual experiences were. What were our first experiences of touching and being touched, the first sexual encounter? Defining sexual desire as the power of self-knowledge and self-love provides a way to speak about it while cautioning girls against the very real dangers of sex. By acknowledging desire we can encourage girls to be prepared for the day when it takes hold of them — and also to distinguish between lust and love. Then, when the culture tells girls to be sexy but not sexual, we will have ways to explain to our daughters that in fact it's normal to *feel* sexual desire but that it's okay to delay acting on this desire by having sex.

# NINE

# Out of the Loop

## GETTING FATHERS INVOLVED

....................❖....................

If we all sat down together to brainstorm an ideal plan for sexuality education, would we develop one in which important male figures in a young girl's life were included? It would seem so natural and obvious, yet dads or male guardians are usually left out of the conversation.

I heard a few stories from daughters and mothers that included their fathers, grandfathers, brothers, husbands, and boyfriends. Only a handful, however, specifically mentioned fathers as a source of emotional support or sexual information. Growing up, Ingrid Shepherd didn't hesitate to go to her dad for questions about sex if her mother wasn't available. However, at some point she noticed a shift in the way she and her father were interacting. For reasons she didn't quite fathom, she felt less comfortable than she had: "I'm still not completely at the same ease with my dad as I am with my mom."

Cindy Gordon's dad made concerted efforts to educate his daughters on how boys think about girls. Stan's openness had a positive impact on his relationship with Cindy, to the point that Cindy said her dad was the one she would go to initially if she ever got into any kind of trouble, including getting pregnant. She recognized, however, that she was the exception: "A lot of my friends would be like, 'I would never tell my dad, he would flip.' "

Living separately from their daughters did not necessarily preclude fathers' involvement. Mel Robbins, who lived in the Midwest, had been divorced from Mary for a number of years, but Vicki and Mel remained in close touch. "It was never really hard," she reflected, "because I know my father will always be there for me no matter what. I know he loves me . . . and I know he's there for me to talk to. My father still tells me you have to love the person before you have sex with him."

The close relationships these three girls described with their fathers, however, were the exceptions. A few, like Katrina and Ruth, viewed their fathers as important figures but did not discuss emotional topics with them. After moving in with her dad during the academic year, Katrina decided he had little idea about what went on in the world of teenagers. "In his work as a high school principal, he obviously sees teens," she said. "So he has to know *something* that's going on, but you know, when you think about your father knowing what you're doing, it's kind of upsetting." Angela Parks rarely spoke with her father and considered him "irrelevant" to her life, while Tiffany Henderson also had an uneasy relationship with her dad. Her mother worried: "I don't want her to get involved with just some guy who won't be good for her to make up for what she doesn't have at home."

Whether the household had two parents or just one, it was rare for a girl to mention her father as a source of sexual knowledge or as someone who communicated with her about personal issues. This was also true for the mothers' generation. In my survey of sixty mothers, when asked "What role did your father play in your own education about sex?" almost all said their father had had no role. "I lived in fear of my father," reported one, "and would never question him about anything." Another said that her dad "*never* uttered a word about it. . . . My father left all the messy emotional stuff to my mother. He was just the brains of the family."

Only a small percentage of these grown women said their fathers had played a notable role in how they learned about sex and sexuality. Occasionally dads had passed along frank advice or explained the importance of abstinence. One woman commented that her father "only advised me not to sit on boys' laps — it aroused them too much." Some dads made efforts to provide more useful information. "When I was little," reminisced one woman, "my dad would answer questions about the difference between boys and girls. Then when I was older, he would interpret adolescent boys to me." Another mother explained, "After my mother died in my early teens, my father was left to answer my questions, and he answered everything I asked him as best he could, but his ears used to get red as he answered."

Ninety-eight percent of these women said that their own fathers were not involved in their sex education, yet almost all (94 percent) of the mothers believed it was important that today's fathers be included. Where dads can be most helpful, they thought, is in telling their girls about how men think and behave and what they want in a relationship. One mother said she thought fathers could "teach daughters to differentiate the true thoughts from the lies boys throw out to increase sexual success." Another stated, "The best thing a father can do is be a good role model."

Some moms believed daughters would benefit greatly if dads explained some of the potential ill effects and dangers of sexual activity. "I think [fathers] should talk with them about love, desire, passion and responsibility. I wish fathers' roles were equal to mothers'," one woman lamented. Another felt that "before girls are sexually active, fathers should tell daughters what men think because men don't think like us."

## The Roots of Distance and Discomfort

Of course, not all fathers will feel comfortable answering specific questions about sex, and girls may share their discomfort. One evening after dinner, Ruth and her sisters were reading in the family room with their parents. Ruth's sister, who was perusing *Seventeen* magazine, looked up and asked, "What's masturbation?" As Ruth told it, "My dad just like zoomed out of the room as fast as he could, and my mom made this gasping sound."

What is it that makes many men so uncomfortable talking about sexuality with their girls? Looking at father-daughter communication in general sheds some light. It would appear, based on several studies, that most dads are only peripherally involved in communicating with their girls about any personal matters. As a girl approaches adolescence, her father not only "pale[s] beside the mother" as a confidant but becomes "someone [girls] would positively avoid, the person they would turn to last." It is not that dad is so much feared or distrusted; he simply is thought to look "ridiculously inept" on personal issues even if he is perceived as the authoritative figure in the household.[1]

Fathers' interactions with their children also tend to decrease as they get older, particularly in the case of daughters. In one study of fifty-five adolescents between the ages of ten and fourteen, adolescent daughters and fathers held significantly different views about the amount of time they spent together. If, for example, a father was clearing the table and the daughter was reading a book in the other room, a father would check this as "spending time together," whereas the daughter did not. Even when dads and daughters agreed on the amount of time spent together, mothers were present for a good deal of it. All in all, dads spent about 3.6 percent of waking hours per day with their girls without moms around.[2]

When fathers are present, they may find it difficult to feel entirely comfortable sharing their male perspective with their daughters. "The biggest problem with fathers is they don't want to accept that their little girl may lose her virginity," reported one mother. Her perception is backed up by psychiatrist Marianne Goodman: "The best of fathers," she observes, "have trouble coming to terms with their little girl's increasing sexuality and growing into adulthood."[3] It can be disconcerting for a dad to see his soccer-playing daughter shift her interests to flirting with boys at the mall.

Nor are dads always equipped with the tools or language to communicate effectively with girls; many families lack any earlier model or preparation for such discussions. In a recent article entitled "Fatherhood Reconsidered," the authors concluded that until recently, American fathers internalized rules and roles rooted in long-standing cultural values and stereotypes, such as "breadwinner," "provider," "disciplinarian," and "connection with the outside world." And in a men's consciousness-raising group — which itself is a major break with traditional values — fathers talked about feeling called upon to demon-

strate emotional skills for which they had no training. To talk intimately about careers and education with their teenage daughters was
difficult enough. They felt discussion of sexual issues and values
should be left to mothers; both parents viewed moms as having the responsibility for that task as well as the necessary empathy.[4]

Dads' uneasiness can translate to girls getting short shrift in their
sexual education. In a study of twenty-two teenage mothers and in another study that looked specifically at parent-daughter communication
around sexual topics, the contributions of dads were negligible. The
most notable aspect of fathers' involvement, in fact, was their *almost
complete absence* from their children's sex education. Only in the least
intense, most abstract discussions of sex was there communication between dad and daughter.[5]

Watching a teenage daughter's sexuality unfold as she sashays
around the house can be perplexing — and a father knows that all
eyes are on him to see how he will address his daughter's emerging
sexuality. The deep-seated incest taboo lingers in the background of
father–adolescent daughter relationships, and a dad may distance himself because of an unconscious fear that he may become sexually attracted to his daughter.[6] Even if he feels comfortable and confident in
his relationship with her, no dad wants others to misjudge him, thinking the relationship too intimate.

One divorced father, Ethan, recounted a graphic scene of his
daughter's metamorphosis and his own experience with society's wariness about father-daughter relationships. Ethan's ten-year-old daughter, Amanda, spent every other weekend at his house. One Saturday
Amanda called him upstairs. "Come on down here," he called back.
"No," she insisted. "You need to come up." Sensing the urgency in her
voice, Ethan went upstairs. She was in the bathroom and told him to
come in. She pointed to her underwear. "I'm bleeding." Ethan looked.
"I think," he said, "you have just started to menstruate. Just wait here."
From his own bathroom, Ethan grabbed the sanitary napkins that his
ex-wife had left him for just such an occasion and returned with several. Amanda knew what she needed to do, and he told her to come
downstairs when she was done. Afterward they talked for a few min-

utes, and he asked if she wanted to call her mom. Amanda didn't think that was necessary. "I wanted to treat this as something normal, and she seemed very relaxed. We went about the day. That night, in the middle of the night, she woke me up. She woke to discomfort and found blood soaked through the sheet. We puzzled out what to do together, I cleaned up the bed, she cleaned up herself, and the next morning we called for maternal backup."

Ethan was proud that his daughter had felt comfortable enough to call out to him for help and thought he had handled the situation well — until he shared his story at a seminar one day with colleagues in his psychology program. "We were discussing adolescent development. When the discussion focused on girls, the faculty member running the seminar, an older man, said 'That's not a man's business.' I disagreed. I said that for divorced fathers that wasn't always true, and I told the story about my experience with Amanda to make my point."

His colleagues, Ethan said, were appalled. It was clear that they thought he should not have been in a bathroom with his ten-year-old daughter and should not have discussed with her how to deal with her period. "Although no one spoke the word, thoughts of incest were in the air — but they weren't my thoughts," he said. "My relationships with this group have never been the same since I told this story. It made me realize how absolutely dangerous it is for a man to be involved in some of the developmental changes of his daughter, even in the most positive ways. That I am even telling you this story feels like a real risk. There is something wrong about this — and I don't think it is how I responded to my daughter's needs." What disturbed Ethan the most was the presumption that mature men, responsible fathers, were incapable of behaving in parentally appropriate ways without sexual overtones.

Stepping back for a moment, the group's reaction seems misplaced. How else might Ethan have handled this? What was his alternative? Was he not supposed to respond to his daughter's call for help? Such a reaction likely would have been more distressing to Amanda; she had requested her dad's assistance, after all. In fact, Ethan acted as a concerned and supportive parent should, treating

Amanda's period as a natural event. Had he panicked, refused to help, expressed discomfort, or called her mother, among the messages conveyed would have been that this subject was off-limits for men and slightly frightening. Ethan's response was a healthy one and a loving one for Amanda and for him.

When fathers are left out of the loop, girls get a confusing message. On the one hand, it says that sex and sexuality are not normal enough or natural enough to be discussed easily and openly and, on the other, that fathers, and by association men in general, are not adult and sensitive enough to understand the issues or make a useful contribution to the conversation. Most families have traditionally handled the sexual concerns that come with a father-daughter relationship by distancing the father. Although a few fathers do cross the line and sexually abuse their daughters, that is the exception. Nevertheless, the taboo remains very strong and may cause some fathers to be especially cautious when their girls enter puberty.

But how puzzling it must be for a girl who has been used to being daddy's little girl, to snuggling in her father's lap and being tucked in at bedtime, suddenly to find her father pulling away. "You are too big for that now," her mother or father tells her. Too big for family hugs? Too big for paternal love? "It feels like you did something wrong," one teenager explained when talking about how her father started distancing himself.

For divorced dads, dealing with a daughter's emerging adolescence can be even more difficult. We know that many daughters feel detached from their fathers even in intact families, but that detachment is compounded by divorce — and almost 50 percent of all couples in first marriage divorce and an additional 17 percent separate. Though custody laws have shifted in the last few years, and more divorced fathers are assuming the role of primary caretaker, the great majority of children live with their mothers. Judith Wallerstein, an expert on children of divorce, found in her longitudinal study that fewer than one-third of the fathers remained closely involved with their children five years after divorce. In addition, fathers who strive to stay involved initially become increasingly detached over time.[7] Losing such a key relationship is often very hard for a girl.

Many divorced families, however, are beginning to recognize the importance of both parents staying close to their children and are working to ensure the fathers' continued involvement during adolescence. One mother told how she and her ex-husband had worked out the parenting of their children. "For one thing, he lives just half a block away from us, so it makes it easy for the children to drop by and see their dad almost on a daily basis. And he also comes to my home to be with the children." She talked with her ex-husband on the telephone at least once a week about the kids' needs and concerns. Recently, when she felt her daughter was turning a cold shoulder to her concerns about her peer group, she asked her ex-husband to talk to her.

Whatever the roots of fathers' drawing back from adolescent daughters — lack of role modeling and preparation for this role, a pervasive belief that a father should not have a close relationship with his adolescent daughter, concerns around incest, or the logistical and emotional difficulties of divorce and separation — none of these has to be an insurmountable obstacle.

## What Fathers Can Say

When a father or another respected male family member says to a daughter, "You are a terrific young woman, and any man who doesn't appreciate all your good qualities, who puts you down or pushes you to act in ways that are against your good judgment is not worthy of you," he is not only building her self-esteem but giving her appropriately high standards for the men she will seek attachments with. When a dad displays admiration and respect for his teenage daughter and praises her accomplishments, he reinforces her belief that she is "okay."[8] If fathers can go beyond this stage to talk more specifically about the importance of communication, respect, and common values in relationships, girls benefit even more. And when dads feel at ease joining their wives in discussing sexuality and the host of other issues that come up in adolescence, as Ingrid's parents did, they stand to learn a few things. Such conversations are, after all, a two-way street.

Perhaps a first step in bringing fathers into the loop of their adolescent girls' sexuality education is for dads to understand how valuable and life-shaping their approval is. Simply spending time together and acknowledging a daughter's strengths signifies concern and caring. When a father is not available, a grandfather, brother, uncle, stepfather, or family friend can also offer the kind of respectful admiration that helps girls develop a positive sense of themselves.

What girls most especially need from fathers is affection, respect, and open communication. As important as it is to tell them what men want, fathers help daughters even more when they continue to talk with and praise them as they become teenagers. Girls like Ingrid, who envision taking an active role in the world and who note the approval reflected in a father's eyes, are less apt to fall into destructive behaviors than girls who do not receive that approval.

Dads can also give a valuable perspective on the information girls get from boys. Calling on their own pasts, they can offer a window into the adolescent boy's mind. As one mother noted, her husband was "much more scared of extreme behavior and sex and that sort of thing. Because when he was a teenager, he was doing it. . . . He has the male point of view that I don't have . . . so that's good."

Some fathers do not talk easily with their own wives about contraception and pregnancy, emotions and feelings, so it can be hard to explain to a daughter that an important part of love is open, easy communication. For many, it is much easier to take a hard line — "Just don't do it" — and say no more than to run the risk of getting into a lengthier conversation that feels difficult. But how helpful it would be to have both parents acknowledge a teenage girl's newfound interest in boys and talk about ways to handle uncomfortable requests. Girls need to be equipped with the words and skills to remove themselves from awkward situations; dads can lend a hand through this, even through role playing ways to resist peer pressure.

The hard-edged approach of "Just don't do it" rolls all too easily through a teenager's brain. A softer, more sensitive tack is to ask a daughter what conditions she thinks should be in place before a man and woman consider intimacy. Granted, some daughters will be too uncomfortable to engage in this kind of positive discussion. "I do try to talk with my daughter about things like AIDS and boys," one father lamented, "but she just looks at me and says, 'Daaaad, you've told me that a million times. Is there anything new you have to say?' It's a little discouraging." This daughter's response is not unusual: girls are not always going to feign interest in dads' concern. Even so, the strong message is: your dad cares.

Mothers can also encourage paternal participation. When Ruth Rosenbloom's father would comment on a sex-related question raised at dinner, Ruth would sometimes hit the table and say, "I can't believe you're saying this in front of us." But Phyllis wisely supported her husband's participation. When fathers are involved in the education of their daughters from the earliest stages, girls have the advantage of two trusted and reliable people they can approach for consultation and questions.

Betsy and Stan Gordon felt there was a substantial payoff for both parents' being involved in teaching their girls early on about sex. Betsy conscientiously involved her husband in talking with the girls from their preschool years. As Cindy moved into adolescence, they worked together on how to handle issues like Cindy's wanting to study in her bedroom with her boyfriend. "We don't always agree," Betsy said, "but we work it out behind the scenes first." The earlier the family signals that these kinds of discussions are acceptable and comfortable, the greater the chances that a daughter in midadolescence will be open to helpful talk.

## Into the Loop

With the changing roles of both women and men in families over the past thirty years, both the quantity of time fathers spend with their children and the types of interactions and activities in which they engage are changing as well.[9] If in the 1950s, fathers' involvement was restricted to "masculine" roles, in the 1990s it is much broader. Dads don't just toss the ball around and fire up the barbecue. They play Nintendo, go to school plays, stay home on a child's sick day, and even join the PTA.

There is reason to be hopeful. We are seeing more examples of fathers becoming actively involved in their daughters' lives and nurturing a close relationship. An article in one of our local newspapers would have been most unusual a couple of decades ago. It described a special birthday present a divorced father received from his twelve-year-old daughter, who lived with her mother. When he picked up the phone, her first words were "Dad, I've got my period." Reflecting on his daughter's call, he wrote: "No other statement to this day has ever touched me so deeply or meant so much to me. The trust behind it was immense. I was male, I was a parent, I was the 'other parent,' yet she could understand I would want to know, that I would be proud of her menstrual flow into womanhood."[10]

The unease many men experience in discussing emotions, coupled with the fact that mothers generally have better interpersonal skills with their children and are viewed as the family's "sex communicators" have made it difficult for some families to break out of time-worn roles. Either consciously or unconsciously, some mothers may also act in ways that exclude fathers from interacting more closely with their daughters. But it is possible for fathers to maintain a comfortable distance from the intimate details of female adolescent development and still contribute significantly to their daughters' understanding of themselves and of men. Mel Robbins talked to Vicki about the importance of love and commitment in a relationship. Dave Shepherd answered Ingrid's questions about sexuality at every stage of her development. Stan Gordon tried to prepare his girls for dating by sharing his own adolescent experiences. There are ample opportunities for dads to enrich their girls' lives without finding a new language or moving into force fields that feel emotionally precarious.

Fathers can also play another critical role by helping to end the silence that surrounds physical and emotional abuse of women. An incident in my own family many years ago is illustrative of both what fathers might do and how they might do more. I'll never forget the evening when my husband and I were eating dinner with our three adolescent children, and Katherine, then twelve, asked about an article on the front page of the local newspaper concerning an eight-year-old girl who had been raped. My husband made a comment about safety in our community and how upsetting such an event would be for a family. He also mentioned that if anyone ever tried to harm his daughter in any way, he would not stop until he found the person. These were important messages for him to convey and, I supposed, a comfort to Katherine. I thought I didn't need to get involved in the conversation.

But the discussion came to a halt when Katherine asked, "Well, what I want to know is how does a grown man get his penis into an eight-year-old girl's vagina?" My husband, his mouth full of rice, sounded as if he were choking. Jon, the fourteen-year-old, put both hands on the table, pushed his chair back, threw his napkin down as if he had assumed the official referee role of this event, and yelled, "Time out! Whoa! Time out!" Jay, who was eleven, was uncharacteristically speechless. I felt all eyes look my way. "Well," I said, "I think it would be very, very difficult, and I am sure it really hurt this little girl and her vagina was torn and she was bleeding." I have no recollection of the males at the table saying another word.

When Katherine raised the issue of rape at the dinner table, she handed her father a perfect opening to speak from a male point of view to our sons as well as to her about the total unacceptability of sex with force at any age under any circumstance. Rape or attempted rape is not about sex; it is about violence, and even if men traditionally feel constrained in discussing sex, they are not strangers to talking about violence. How many daughters might be spared needless pain if dads could help them understand that if they ever feel they are being threatened, harassed, or harmed in any way, they should come to their parents for guidance and support?

It may have been important for my daughter to know that her father would relentlessly pursue anyone who did her harm, but I think, reflecting on girls who have been raped and have never spoken of it, that it was as important for Katherine to know that the victim would not be blamed. She would be loved and cherished by us no matter what kind of threats or violence others inflicted on her life.

Many of us have learned not to let racist or sexist comments pass as if we condone them. When men protest any form of violence against women, they aid daughters everywhere. To date, this has been a battle fought mainly by women, but it is impossible to win without men's support. Girls who, like Cindy Gordon, understand from both parents that violence is never acceptable in relationships with boys, are more likely to remove themselves from abusive circumstances. In turn, when adolescent girls refuse to tolerate any physical or emotional abuse from their dates, they help to educate teenage boys.[11]

Portraying men as one-dimensional sex-driven creatures creates its own predicament: it sets our girls up to expect nothing more of them. But fathers can give girls insight into boys' behavior and help them become self-assured enough to establish acceptable standards of conduct for the boys they date. A father contributes to his daughter's sexual education when he says, "Look, you can be charmed by a guy's looks or his line or his energy or the attention he pays you, and all that is important, but look behind all that, and make sure you respect the way he leads his life. Look at how he acts with his friends and his family and other adults; look at what he thinks of himself and what he wants to accomplish. Don't even think of becoming involved with any guy who doesn't respect you and doesn't care for your feelings." It's dads who can best explain that young men generally come much later to an appreciation of relationships than young women and that postponing sexual intimacy until after adolescence gives boys time to mature emotionally and girls time to develop the emotional stability for a successful relationship.

Family discussions may be easier than father-daughter conversations. What better way for sons to understand how they are expected to behave with women than to hear their father explaining this to a daughter over dessert? What better way for a daughter to understand men than through the concerned tutelage of her father or uncle or grandfather? If the father cannot convey these messages, it is important that she find positive adult male role models to help her develop high standards for her future partner.

No matter how wise we are as mothers, we can only report from the female perspective. In most cases our daughters are going to fall in love and become intimate with men. Surely it makes sense for the important man in a girl's growing-up years, the man who has unquestionably already shaped her opinions, to participate as she learns to come to terms with her own sexuality and with relationships. Participation by fathers helps girls, and it honors fathers.

# TEN

# Getting It Right

## MATERNAL STRATEGIES

...................... ❧ ......................

W hy is it so hard for so many of us to discuss sex? "I never
talked about it," one mother explained, "because I was never
quite sure what I should say or when I should say it, and by the time
I thought I might be ready, my daughter had stopped talking. . . . I
needed a script." Some of us have inherited our own mothers' discomfort in talking about sex. Sometimes we're uncertain about what to say
— we'd rather say nothing than say the wrong thing. We also find it
very difficult to talk about our feelings related to sexual topics. And at
times even the most outspoken mother wrestles with her thoughts
when a daughter presents her with an unexpected situation.

At a recent dinner party, a mother of a sixteen-year-old poured out
her maternal concern to me. Patricia and her daughter, Nancy, had always had an open and easy relationship, so open that Nancy had admitted to her mother that her boyfriend had broached the subject of
sex. When Nancy told her boyfriend she didn't feel ready for such an
intimate relationship, he had been understanding and respectful. Patricia was proud of Nancy's decision and thought she could rest easy
— until the day she discovered a Victoria's Secret bag under Nancy's
bed when she was cleaning. She peeked inside to find a sexy black
lace bra and matching panties. Immediately she wondered, Did Nancy
and Bill buy these together? Had Bill seen her daughter in these?

Patricia and her husband talked about what to do and decided not to say anything. But she kept thinking about the lingerie and what it might mean. Now, at the dinner party, she confessed, "I thought seeing Nancy through adolescence was going to be relatively easy, but it doesn't seem so easy now. What should I do?" Here was one of those situations not covered in any basic handbook on sex. Tied up in this mother's discovery were issues of trusting and of not wanting to intrude. I wished that I could tell her to look in the index under "Victoria's Secret" in some book to find the precise advice for dealing effectively with her situation.

As we know all too well, there is no single "right" response to most questions concerning sex and sexuality. And when women agree on the right response to an issue, they often choose different strategies for presenting it, or their daughters require different approaches. Yet despite these variations, the common denominator to effective communication is open, two-way communication. Silence often begets more problems and anxieties.

Girls will learn about menstruation, intercourse, and reproduction whether or not we say one word (the accuracy of the information is another matter). With any selection from a pile of good books, we can present all the reproductive mechanics she needs. But if anything becomes clear from the stories of mother-daughter communication, it is the importance of having an ongoing dialogue with our daughters, of piecing together the nuts and bolts for them, and of broadening the context in which the facts are placed. A wide-ranging dialogue is critical for a host of reasons, but four main factors were highlighted by the interviews:

- ❋ Not talking sends its own message, one that is very likely to cause daughters to feel confused about their sexual thoughts and feelings. What are they to surmise if we talk with them about most other aspects of their development but remain mute about sex?

- ❋ With sex, facts are not enough. Young people are in the process of developing their own framework of values, and by talking about our feelings, our beliefs, the culture of our family and our community, and the moral code by which we live, we give our daughters a richer context to make sense of the facts. We should leave room for their evolving belief systems in our discussions.

❀ Teens are bombarded with sexual information and imagery from television, books, movies, music, and countless other sources. We need to bring into sharper focus the often inaccurate portrayals of sex and relationships that the media project. We put our girls at risk if we hand over the sex education of our daughters to these sources that bear no personal connection to us.

❀ When girls misunderstand the appeal — and possible repercussions — of becoming sexually engaged, the consequences may be difficult and sometimes painful. An important part of parental responsibility is to provide our children with the information, skills, and resources they need to guard against physical and emotional harm.

Sex is not a discrete body of knowledge that can be isolated from the rest of life. Talking about sex implies talking about relationships, self-esteem, feminism and femininity, gender differences, marriage and maternity, men and paternity. On a broader canvas, it means discussing values and expectations. Realizing that "sex" is really only one part of sex education can help us to seize opportunities for candid discussion. For Nancy's mother, the potential conversation was not about lingerie but about Nancy's normal pull toward sexual exploration and about the kinds of conditions that should be in place for her to become sexually involved.

## The Wisdom of Hindsight

Enriched by the knowledge of the mothers and daughters I spoke with, I wish I could relive my relationship with my daughter during her adolescence. I would say more and believe less that I could determine Katherine's decisions. I would understand that whatever guidance I gave her, she would ultimately make her own decisions. I'd also weigh more carefully the types of messages I conveyed, both spoken and unspoken. I'd try to emphasize issues of self-esteem and discuss my hopes for her as a young woman, while still giving credence to the dangers of disease and emotional distress. Most important, though, I would make a concerted effort to understand that my daughter was becoming a sexual being and to embrace that part of her as much as her intellectual capacity, her temperamental strengths and weaknesses, her musical gifts and athletic proclivities. I'd try to help her understand her sexuality in the context of our family's values and religious beliefs.

It all sounds so easy in hindsight, but in truth, I believe today I would be less fearful of saying too much to my adolescent. I wouldn't hesitate, for instance, to talk about any aspect of sexuality, no matter how peculiarly it struck me, if my daughter broached it — or if it appeared in the newspaper or on television. I would use a variety of strategies to ensure that topics were addressed. Incredibly, I never talked with Katherine about contraception, and now I cannot imagine neglecting this subject. I would speak specifically about contraceptives and sexually transmitted diseases while emphasizing that sex must always be seen as one aspect of a relationship. I would encourage her participation by being a better listener.

Looking back, I realize my efforts to educate Katherine were inspired by a fear of failing to convey to my daughter all the standard messages I thought mothers must impart absolutely, without taking into account the nuances of sex and relationships. I wanted to be sure Katherine knew what was "right" out of an overwhelming desire to prevent anything from going wrong. I was confused and frustrated about what role I should assume in these talks, and I found it difficult to broach some topics. If Katherine were a teenager today, I would probably still feel uncomfortable, but I would know how important it was to share my knowledge and feelings with her. I would also seek support and ideas from other mothers and look for forums for mothers and daughters to discuss sexual topics.

If today I found a bag of sexy lingerie under my teenage daughter's bed, I probably would have some of the initial reactions of Nancy's mother. But then, after some reflection, I hope I could say to my daughter, "Let's talk about this. It tells me you are feeling very feminine and womanly, and that probably means you are thinking a lot about desire and sexuality. I know you need your private space to sort through your own feelings, but it's such a confusing time — for me as well as for you. Can we talk about it, because I know I'm feeling the need to talk?"

Revisiting how we nurtured our girls through other aspects of growing up might offer some reassuring lessons for mothers of adolescents. When Katherine was old enough to cross the street alone, I worried. When she wanted to go to the movies without adults, I was uncomfortable. When I had to let her ride in cars with teenage drivers and then when she drove herself, of course I worried. And when Katherine started to look and act like a woman, I was even more concerned and confused about what I should or should not say.

But we eventually let our children cross the street, go to the movies, and move into the world, because we understand the importance of letting them learn to take care of themselves. We permit them to drive, even if our hearts are pushing out of our chests, and we do all that we can to ensure their safety. We make them drive around the block before we let them drive around the neighborhood, and only reluctantly do we permit them onto the highways. We teach them to wear their seat belts, and we drum into their heads never to drive with someone who has had too much to drink. "Call home any time of the night, and we will come for you, no questions asked," we told our children over and over. Sensible fears about the dangers of driving impel most parents to tell their children as much as possible about driving and safety. So why is it that the perils of sexual intimacy don't similarly lead us to tell our daughters everything we know?

"Sex is private and sex is mysterious. Too much talk takes away the mystery and magic" are sentiments expressed by more than a few mothers. Yet isn't it also true that no matter how many springtimes we watch unfold, the new season is still delicious to behold? No matter how many weddings we attend, we still feel a lump in our throat when the bride walks down the aisle? No matter how many babies we hold, each one is still a wonder. Talking about sex can't possibly take away its mystery.

## Following a Daughter's Lead

Many of us remember the "Big Talk," when our mothers sat us down and, perhaps with an illustrated book explained the Facts of Life. Though that is still a viable approach, a more effective strategy for most mothers and daughters today is having several shorter, informal conversations in which more and more information is discussed. When daughters ask, mothers — and fathers, too — should strive to answer. Rather than telling a girl she is too young to understand the answer to her questions, we can aim to answer in a way that makes sense for her age and development. During the preschool and early school-age years, we can answer questions simply without fretting about elaboration. A satisfactory reply to the question "Where do babies come from?" might be "They come from inside the mother's tummy, where they grow from a tiny egg to a tiny baby." If she wants to know more, trust that she will initiate more conversation. A mother's willingness to answer questions about sex will establish a daughter's trust that it is all right to ask them.

Mothers can easily make the mistake of waiting "until my daughter is old enough to need to know." The ideal time to begin to talk in detail is when our daughters show the first signs of puberty. With some girls now becoming prepubescent as early as age seven or eight, they are often ready to learn about anatomy and biology long before we think they are. Menarche creates a wonderful opportunity for mothers and daughters — and fathers and daughters — to talk at length about a girl's transformation. This may also set the tone for future conversations. A daughter's distinctive developmental readiness, not some chart in a book, should shape the conversation.

As we have seen, the course of adolescent development gives us hints about what to expect and when to expand the level of discussion. Because it is natural for girls to begin to pull away in their midteens, talking early permits mothers to speak freely and establish a close connection before girls embark on the harried arc of adolescence.

## Being Open and Accessible

When a mother is open in talking about sex, it generally sets her daughter at ease. By her comments, questions, responses, and body language, a mother signals that she is comfortable — or that she isn't but hopes her daughter will be. Some mothers balk at the notion of sitting on the sofa with their daughters and discussing the details of intercourse, masturbation, or oral sex. Even if we hesitate or blush when mentioning such terms, mothers can still contribute enormously to a daughter's sexual education by talking generally about what constitutes a mature sexual relationship and how women can achieve their goals in such a relationship. A dialogue about motherhood and the circumstances necessary for a woman to be a good mother or a chat about self-sufficiency and being able to work and provide for oneself before tackling the job of caring for others can help point the way for wise decision-making down the road.

Encouraging daughters to talk with other women as well can be an effective means of compensating for our own hesitancies. Estelle Brown knew that her sister was a reliable resource for Sam; Melinda found great comfort in talking with her aunt. Perhaps a sister, a best friend, or a daughter's friend's mother would be willing to step into the role of consultant.

Not all daughters respond warmly to mothers' attempts to talk, but that isn't necessarily a criticism of a mom's communication style. Some girls need more space or more privacy; some are not prepared to talk when we think they should be. Still others just roll their eyes when we try to instigate conversation. Mothers cannot force their daughters to engage in conversation about sex, nor should we try; but we can let girls know, both directly and indirectly, that we are always available and interested in talking. It can help to say at the right moment, *before* a confrontation begins, something along these lines: "Look, we may not always agree. What is important to me is that we can always talk. When I think you are wrong, of course, I am going to let you know, because that's my job as a mother. But I want you to talk to me about why you think I am off base if you do. We each have different perspectives. I know from experience things you don't know, but you may see things in ways that I don't — and what's important is that we talk. That's how we each learn."

In these one-way mother-to-daughter messages, a daughter may not appear to be paying much attention. Yet as the girls at Nottingham and Jefferson told me, they often are searching for answers and are still reading the nuances of our spoken language and our body language. Alma Parks and Gerry Valentia held fast to the notion that their girls would absorb information through osmosis, even if their daughters looked disinterested. It's important that we, as mothers, as carefully and as gently as we can, continue to converse with our daughters and encourage them to speak with other adult women with whom they feel comfortable.

## Valuing Candor

Being honest with our daughters doesn't mean we must divulge our deepest secrets. Indeed, most daughters don't care to know or think about their mothers as sexual beings. If they do ask questions that seem too personal, it's fine to say, "I want us to be able to talk about any subject in general. What goes on between your father and me, however, is personal, just as what will go on between you and the person you love will be personal." If pressed, a mom might add, as one mother did when her daughter inquired if she engaged in oral sex, "I believe that if two adult people who have a commitment to each other and have demonstrated real care and concern for each other are both comfortable with some aspect of love-making, then it's okay. If one of them is not comfortable, then it's not okay."

Mothers who themselves were sexually active in high school will sometimes advise their daughters, "Nice girls don't have sex with boys." But *they* were nice girls and they had sex, so they know that nice girls do. An alternative is to explain that girls often feel the urge to experience sexual intimacy with a boy and then explore the reasons why, from a mother's vantage point, she might not condone it.

Adolescent girls are bound to follow some course we've advised against, and some will cross that line for sex. Diane Early claimed she was unaware that Melinda was intimately involved with her boyfriend. Mothers may find some comfort in keeping themselves in the dark but that is not a good basis for understanding our girls. Melinda's decision to be sexually active could have provided an opportunity for mother-daughter talk about her feelings for this boy and her long-range hopes for the relationship. It became, instead, an unspoken barrier between them.

## Talking in Ways That Work for Adolescents

The line between constructive repetition and nagging is a delicate one, easy to cross. Nagging, that constant reminding that carries with it negative judgment and the implication of guilt, is usually counter-productive. On the other hand, it can be helpful to revisit old topics with our daughters. If a mother realizes that her daughter is contemplating becoming sexually active, that's the time to find a story that leads to a discussion about contraceptives rather than retreating or re-iterating the virtues of abstinence.

Many daughters report that their mothers never discussed certain topics with them, while mothers have explicit recollections of raising those very topics. It's possible that the timing or presentation of the message made it difficult for the girl to recall her mother's point. Moms are not always effective couriers for their messages, and daughters will screen out information they are not ready to receive. But one lesson the girls at Jefferson and Nottingham drove home is this: teens need to feel they are being heard before they can hear us. We constantly have to ask ourselves: Am I listening to her? Do I let her know I'm listening by giving her time to speak and allowing her the space to say what she wants? Am I absorbing what she's saying without making instant interpretations or passing judgment? Do I make eye contact and use the skills of active listening? Betty Graham referred to "those cute little listening tricks" she turned to "almost out of desperation" in her efforts to improve her interactions with thirteen-year-old Camille. Before, when Camille shared a problem, Betty would launch into suggestions on how to handle it. "I've had to turn that off. I'm far more careful, and I try to do more listening." Another mother reported that her communication with her teen improved when she began "holding my breath and counting to ten before speaking."

Sometimes a mother means well, but her maternal suggestions come across as niggling and intrusive. One mother, for instance, criticized her daughter's clothing and asked repeatedly where she was going and what she was doing. She reminded her daughter that being responsible meant cleaning her room and doing her chores. To her mind, these messages were a mother's duty, but they annoyed her daughter. In her eyes, her mother's comments added up to constant criticism, and as a result she pulled further and further away.

When my children were little I thought all mothers should have honorary membership in the Teamsters' union because we did so much hauling, lifting, and driving. But as we progress to mothering adolescents, we ought to be awarded honorary psychology degrees, because we must learn to think so carefully about our own patterns and those of our children. Communication with adolescents must be tailored to their needs — which do not always dovetail with our own. Alma Parks wanted to spend time talking with her daughters while they all cleaned house on the weekends. She thought this was an efficient blend of accomplishing household tasks and being together, but it provoked so much controversy that Angela moved in with her grandmother for a year. Once Alma understood that Angela would rather have a job than clean house and that Angela was still a responsible adolescent even if she hated vacuuming, they were able to stop fighting and begin talking.

As girls chart their course through adolescence, they frequently take extreme positions and find fault with moms' every word. But when we convey, by our actions and words, the message "No, you cannot say this, think this, feel this," we do little to foster self-esteem or critical thinking skills. It is hard to see girls trying on new ideas that we feel uncomfortable with — and it is our responsibility to make our feelings clear and set limits on their behavior. This is quite different, however, from telling girls what they *should* feel or think.

When we refuse to listen to our daughters and talk only about what we wish and fear for them, we suggest that we have little confidence in their ability to make good decisions. When mothers trust, listen, and reassure their daughters that they are learning good judgment and making good decisions, girls are more likely to be responsible and responsive. And when they aren't responsible, when they make mistakes and use faulty judgment, we also need to be there to help them find their way back. Columnist Ellen Goodman once wrote, wisely, "Every one of us crosses the time zone of our kids' adolescence with our eyes open and our fingers crossed. We want to keep them safe and get them out on their own. They want to be emancipated and protected. There's no trickier time. But if there's any hedge against trouble, it's in building a relationship of trust — not blind trust but reasonable trust. And when it's broken, rebuilding it."[1]

## Seizing the Opportunities

I will always remember Alma Parks looking at me with fire in her eyes and saying, "Sex is everywhere, so why should I hush my mouth?" She was right; sex *is* everywhere, and we have ample material for conversation starters. Joan Rankin turned to *Beverly Hills 90210* and other popular programs to stimulate discussions about values. Estelle Brown used Magic Johnson's admission that he was HIV-positive to talk with Samantha about AIDS and the importance of using condoms. Gerry Valentia made her kitchen a comfortable environment for teen talk and gleaned the goings-on of her girls' world from their conversations. Many mothers commented on the effectiveness of a drive in the car for stimulating conversation. "She can't walk away," one mother noted, "or go to her room and close the door, but she doesn't have to make eye contact with me." Daughters can talk from the back seat and mothers from the front without ever having to face off on the subject at hand.

If driving edges some girls into conversation, the late-night hours lead others to open up, often when they return from parties or dates.

During my daughter's adolescence, I always struggled to stay awake when she was out late because she would share details at midnight that would have faded by the next morning. Other mothers reported similar moonlighting duties.

When our daughters tell us of rejection, disappointment, or deceit, we hurt with them and for them. Encouraging them to cope head on with life's disappointments can help them to handle deftly the larger ones later on. A bad grade on one test isn't a summary judgment on intelligence. Likewise, rejection by a boyfriend doesn't mean a lifetime of being alone. When we praise a young woman for her accomplishments and continually reinforce the notion that she should never tolerate anything but respect and thoughtfulness from a young man — or anyone else, for that matter — we contribute to building self-esteem.

Still, busy working parents like Marian Henderson may despair at finding the time or the overlap with their girls' schedules to have intimate chats. That's when it falls to parents to *create* an opportunity, no matter how small. What is our daughter's world like? Do we know what other girls her age are wearing, doing, saying? Who are her friends? Though finding time can seem a herculean task, if a mother can get time off to go on a school field trip once a semester or volunteer at school one afternoon a month, she will get an invaluable look at her daughter's life. Being the scorekeeper for the girls' volleyball team or driving the van to the team game are all activities that put us in close proximity with our daughters and their peers.

Eating together is another way to bring a teenager into our orbit. Regular family meals, with the television off, the phone answering machine on, and everyone at the table, create an excellent environment for wide-ranging conversation. Cooking together — baking cakes, cookies, or pizza for a party after a high school football game can also provide opportunities for talking. Some families like to arrange a time for one child and one parent to go off together apart from the hustle-bustle of the family routine. It might be a once-a-month Sunday breakfast at a local coffee shop, a weekly visit to a favorite Chinese restaurant. Whatever the choice, it can make a daughter feel special.

## Stressing Relationships

Perhaps the most important lesson I have taken from my work with adolescent girls and moms is that talk about sex needs to be grounded in the context of relationships. Our daughters struggle with how they want to see and be seen in the adult world by their parents, their peers, other mentoring adults, the opposite sex, and God. The wish for a love relationship typically holds greater sway in girls' minds than the biology of desire.

To bring questions about relationships into clear focus, girls first need to feel comfortable with and have confidence in themselves. The first step, then, is helping them build self-esteem, which comes from believing they are lovable and understanding that there are adults who care for them. When a young girl sets a goal and accomplishes it, she flexes her esteem muscles; when she is praised — not gratuitously but legitimately — for her efforts, again her confidence grows. Helping daughters develop their athletic, artistic, and academic competencies is part of this esteem-building process. When the inevitable difficulties arise, guiding them to develop their own solutions rather than trying to "save them" by solving their problems promotes maturity.

Our daughters are learning to laugh and to work, to discipline themselves and forgive themselves — and they learn their lessons most readily from us. If parents set standards so high that their children keep missing the mark, they may decide to give up rather than try harder. On the other hand, if our expectations are too low, there is little gratification in meeting them. Every girl needs to experience some successes in her early adolescence, and when these are not readily attainable, parents ought to try to create opportunities that will yield successes. In the same vein, every girl needs a few struggles to establish that the world doesn't always provide what we want — but not so many as to break her spirit.

As it becomes more difficult in midadolescence to address sexuality head on, the focus of parental involvement can switch to informal conversations about relationships. Just as the media offer abundant references to sex, so too they illustrate a whole gamut of relationship issues. These "props" can lead to lively family discussions. Even a brief comment can be effective — sometimes more effective than a long "lesson." For example, watching a movie in which a young woman had sex with a man she hardly knew, a mother told her sixteen-year-old daughter: "How foolish of that young woman to risk her body and her heart with a person she has only known a day, when there is so little to gain and so much to risk." A powerful view conveyed in little time.

## Trusting Our Instincts

Trust maternal instinct. If we sense in our gut that something is amiss with our daughter, we ought to respect that inner voice. Mothers are not private investigators or district attorneys. We needn't amass evidence and assemble case histories to argue a point. One of the prerogatives of being mothers is that we are allowed to say, "Hold on, something doesn't feel right here. I'm getting vibrations that we need to talk." Of course, just because we express our concern doesn't guarantee that our daughter will reveal what's wrong, but it's a necessary start.

If a daughter is befriending peers who are likely to get her into trouble or is making dangerous choices, it may be that she has a poor self-image or is searching for something to keep her engaged. A parent can suggest some different after-school or community activities she might be interested in. At the other end of the spectrum, if a girl's malaise is tied to something happening in the home, family counseling may be useful. Families function as interconnected networks, and the actions and attitudes of one family member affects everyone.

Girls in junior high often sound as though they are absolutely, positively sure of their world, completely intransigent in their positions, and determined to berate whatever we suggest. While it is important to respect their ideas and listen carefully to their positions, it is not necessary, in the end, to agree with them. Most mothers are wiser than most thirteen-year-olds, no matter how many times we falter. We can't be afraid to have a disappointed daughter shout that she hates us and never wants to see us again because we acted like a responsible parent.

On the other hand, we must remain committed to searching for approaches that favor conversation instead of conflict to resolve problems. The forbidden, we all know, can become the most desirable. One mother remembered with amusement how her parents handled a beau of hers whom they disliked: "He was a very sexy guy, but he didn't have good judgment, good manners, or good sense. My parents insisted on including him in all kinds of family events. We'd go to a nice restaurant and they would make me bring him. They'd never mention his table manners, but they knew we all noticed. They would ask him questions over dessert and let him fumble around for answers. At first, of course, I felt very protective of him, but after a while it was hard not to see what my parents saw. He ended up falling hard for my parents, while I lost interest in him."

## Talking about Desire and the Decision to Have Sex

As one mom acknowledged, despite her best intentions, she worried about the day her daughter "just got that look in [her] eye" for sex. All of us can surely recollect situations in which we were seduced by desire, but how many of us feel at ease speaking forthrightly about its pull? It is, unquestionably, one of the most perplexing topics for discussion, as these mother-daughter pairs attested. We might say we believe there is something very special about waiting to have intercourse with a husband; we might express the belief that mature women may be ready for sex before they are married but that during high school emotional maturity lags behind physical maturity. Or we may wish to help our daughters define the circumstances necessary for sexual intimacy. Certainly women exhibit great variety in the ways they address desire, and we can only share with our daughters what makes sense for us and why.

Figuring out desire in all its complexity is a slow and perplexing business for many girls. In the process, some girls may jump in simply to be done with the question: "Do I or don't I?" One gift we can give our daughters is an appreciation for the importance of making decisions based on their internal needs and values rather than just on the external situation.

Katrina wished for a checklist to help her decide when she would be ready for sexual intimacy. The easiest response is "when you are married," but we know this answer will fail to serve a majority of our daughters today. As more and more women postpone marriage until their late twenties, the virtues, both physical and emotional, of abstinence may become more difficult for young women to appreciate. Sexual intimacy, the girls I spoke with understood, brought responsibilities. It demanded emotional and physical readiness, a partner who was caring and respectful, and an inner certainty — all of which resist convenient scheduling.

Many mothers and girls have asked me, "So, when is it okay for girls to become sexually active?" They seem eager to have a specific age delineated, perhaps a specific day that they can mark on a calendar. I wish it were so easy. Of course, there is no "right" or simple answer to this question, because it hinges so much on each individual girl, her past experiences, her current relationship, and a host of other unquantifiable characteristics. As a health care professional, I am aware that many girls do not develop the emotional and intellectual maturity for sex until they are in their late teens or early twenties, and it is my professional opinion that it is best for girls to postpone intercourse until they have reached this level of maturity. Although each girl will make her decisions individually, I do think we can give a young woman some clear cautions about signs that she is *not* yet prepared for sexual activity:

❋ If she is not ready to go to a doctor and take responsibility for her own contraception

❋ If she does not feel comfortable discussing sexuality with her proposed partner

* If her proposed partner is not willing to use contraception himself in every sexual encounter
* If she is filled with doubt about what she is doing
* If she feels ashamed about what she is doing
* If she is not willing to be honest with her partner and is not sure of his honesty with her
* If she and her partner have not discussed what they would do if she were to become pregnant
* If she doesn't like her partner's friends and doesn't trust his judgment
* If she has any suspicion that her partner has been sexually involved with others and has not been tested for AIDS
* If she needs alcohol or drugs to make her feel relaxed enough for sex
* If she is responding to someone else's needs and not her own

Even if a young woman feels certain that she is in a loving and caring relationship, knows about contraception and STDs, and has none of the reservations on the above checklist, she still may not possess the emotional sophistication to reach a wise decision about sex. Moreover, a teenage girl can't possibly have the wide-ranging perspective of a slightly older woman, who can compare her current relationship to some others. Too many times I have had a girl tell me how she was certain she had discovered love and instead had gotten pregnant. It can seem to an adolescent, in the rush of emotion, as though a high school sweetheart is the be-all and end-all, the guy she will marry, so why not do it all now? But the majority of women do not marry their high school sweethearts. Rather, they have several different relationships before settling on the one that feels right because it is committed and loving.

But I also know as a counselor that many girls do choose to become sexually active in adolescence, and they don't appear to be suffering irreparable harm. More than half of our teenage girls have sex by the time they are eighteen.[2] To say that there is no "okay time" for this group defies reality and suggests that a majority of these girls will meet with harmful outcomes. Adolescent girls are having sex and will continue to do so. As a counselor, I try to provide as much information as girls need to determine for *themselves* when the "right time" will be. As Ingrid Shepherd said, "Before I can make a decision I need to know who believes what and why. If I can get someone who believes it's fine to have sex, I'll ask them why. And I'll listen to those reasons and then I'll go to my own parents or someone else who believes you shouldn't, and I'll say, Why? And then I'll think about those reasons — you just have to have a lot of information."

The decision to become sexually active is ultimately an "adult" one. I use this term loosely, just as we do in other areas of society. To drive, you have to be sixteen; to vote, you have to be eighteen; in most states, you have to be twenty-one to drink. We all know that some seventeen-year-olds are more mature than twenty-year-olds, so to try to define an age criterion for sexual activity seems about as helpful as saying, "Just don't do it." But we also know that many adolescent girls are quick to judge themselves as "adults" and are probably naive about the nuances of a fully developed relationship. Mothers can help sort through these considerations by asking whether we consider our girls young adults and whether our daughters agree — about themselves *and* their partners. Such a conversation would seem to me more useful than an age criterion in helping girls determine when it is "okay" to have sex.

Some daughters may express an attraction to other girls. This can be a natural part of adolescence, and a mother can save her daughter enormous pain and self-doubt by opening the door to discussion and listening to her voice. Mothers play a critical role in reaffirming their girl's sense of self, especially as their sexuality unfolds.

We want our girls to know that sexuality will be with them all their lives, that they needn't be impatient to experience sex. The wiser and more confident they become and the more discriminating they are in choosing partners, the more likely it is that their sexual experiences will be positive.

## Some Practical Strategies

Many mothers I spoke with wanted a quick checklist of the most popular strategies for communicating effectively about sex and sexuality with their girls. Though mothers will no doubt add to and shape this list to their own needs, what follows are some strategies that have worked well for other mothers and daughters:

* *Use books and magazines.* Don't wait until it's time for a "big talk" to search out books about sex. Even before girls enter puberty, moms can begin to review texts to find the words and approaches that feel comfortable. If a daughter prefers to read something on her own, ask if she would let you share it with her. Perhaps you never had this experience with your mom and it would mean a great deal to talk about these things with her. If she is already a teen and you want to forge better communication, you might read parts of books or magazine articles aloud together. Pick up some of the new teen magazines.

* *Arrange a visit with a physician.* By midadolescence, girls ought to know how to contact health resources when necessary. Look for a doctor who sees adolescents in his or her practice. You might ask other mothers for recommendations for a pediatrician, a doctor who specializes in adolescent medicine, an internist, or a gynecologist. Visit the doctor with your daughter and make it clear to the doctor and your daughter that she is free to call or visit with any question. If mothers feel comfortable, their daughters can accompany them for a gynecological exam.

* *Help your daughter know her body.* Adolescence is the time for a girl to begin to develop comfort and familiarity with her body. As she approaches puberty, give her a diagram of the female anatomy that names and describes the parts of the genitalia. Suggest that one day when she is alone, she take a mirror, look at her vagina, and identify all of its parts. While she may be shocked by the suggestion, she'll also know that her mother thinks the vagina, clitoris,

and vulva are not mysterious and unknowable "things" but important parts of her anatomy.

* *Preview the products.* Early in her adolescence, while the conversation still feels general and not specific, go to the drugstore and look at the feminine hygiene and contraception products together. By standing in public with her and looking at these items, mothers send the message that menstruation and contraception are topics that can be discussed. A family's faith or values may lead a mother to recommend against sexual activity and thus contraception before marriage, and this view can be addressed in the context of what is on the shelves — and what is not. Ask your daughter whether contraception was discussed in her health or sex education class at school.

* *Build in time for talk.* Doing something together that you and your daughter enjoy provides an unstructured time for talking. It could be jogging or joining an exercise class, making a quilt, going on a hiking trip, trying out ten chocolate recipes, refinishing a bedroom bureau, volunteering at a food bank, planting a vegetable garden, or shopping for school clothes and topping it off with lunch or dinner. Conversation comes more easily when our daughters can just fall into it rather than feel as if they have been assigned a moment of intimacy.

* *Bring others into the conversation.* If talking one on one is difficult, mothers can turn to groups with other girls who are moving into adolescence. Your religious group, friends, a girl's organization, or a mother-daughter book club may provide such chat sessions. Some middle schools and junior high schools have begun to organize mother-daughter discussion groups. Such a group could invite a health educator to speak or have a series of guest speakers: a gynecologist, a psychologist who works with adolescents, a sex educator, a sports coach, a nutritionist, or a counselor for gay and lesbian teens.

Work with your husband or partner to introduce conversation at the dinner table or around the television if that feels comfortable. Encourage both immediate and extended family members to speak with your daughter. Some parents may want only their own views on sexuality to be heard, but it helps young women become more confident when they hear different views and understand that consensus is a relative term, that a girl must determine what is right for herself.

❋ *Keep a reference book about sex sitting in an easily visible place.* Store a book you like in a place where anyone in the family can pull it down and refer to it when there is a question.

❋ *Focus on family values.* Few teenagers reward parents with complete acceptance of their values, because adolescence is the natural time to test out independent views. The challenge for parents is to encourage adolescents to articulate their perceptions and to consider them in the context of the family's value system.

## Wonder

Sex is amazing. It is different for everyone. It is different with different people and even with the same person. Words cannot describe the sensations and feelings that two people who love and respect each other can create together. These can be completely grasped only in the moment. Little girls often tell their mothers how disgusting sex sounds when it is first described to them. The mystery is that something that seems quite odd in the abstract is so universally desired in the flesh. We need not fear that telling our daughters about sex — about the whole nine yards that Pauline Dickinson says they need to know — will keep girls from its wonder and uniqueness. Rather, we can help daughters delay their sexual explorations if we openly recognize the reality of physical desire but explain that sex is also an activity of the mind. If we can talk with our girls about sexual desire, about men and women and relationships, about our hopes and fears and theirs, too, and about the lines of danger and desire along which adolescents dance, then we stand a better chance of having our daughters postpone sexual intimacy and choose the right time to move forward sexually. In the process of talking, we will be letting our daughters know that the transformation from girlhood to womanhood is normal, natural, and desirable. This positive approach leads to self-confidence, self-esteem, and positive feelings for the future. Adolescents are going to make their own sexual decisions no matter what we say or how we say it, but we can help prepare them to make those decisions responsibly.

# Beyond the Family

## INVOLVING THE COMMUNITY

Sheila McIveney is a very good swimmer. Today, at fifty-three, she swims five miles or more every week with ease. Swimming has become a favorite pastime, but her interest began early: as a young girl, her mother introduced her to swimming in a backyard wading pool. Her father, she says, taught her how to put her head "all the way under." Later she took swimming lessons at the YMCA and swam with friends at the community pool. They taught her to dive, do the butterfly, and make flip turns. In middle school and high school, she was on the swim team and attended swimming clinics; in college, coaches and supportive peers helped her to refine her style and build self-confidence. Not all of Sheila's coaches took the same approach to competitive swimming, but she listened to everybody and figured out a style that worked for her. Her parents were there for all her important meets; whether she won or lost, she says, they were ready with encouragement and understanding.

What's swimming got to do with sex? A simple metaphor really: how Sheila learned to be a good swimmer is not far from how I believe girls should learn about sex and sexuality. The first lessons are learned at home, but as girls grow under their parents' oversight, they also need support and guidance from others in the community. Right now our daughters receive some community input through sex education classes, but the gestures of community institutions pale in comparison to the "information" spewed out by television, movies, and the other media. No one I know has said that they felt these media resources teach in a good way.

Most parents and teens join educators, adolescent development experts, and youth advocates in supporting strong community-based sex education. In fact, between 80 and 90 percent of parents want sexuality education taught in America's schools. An even higher percentage want their children to learn about safe sex as a means of preventing AIDS. Parents have always needed support and assistance from the community in all aspects of child rearing, from pediatricians to daycare, from babysitters to elementary school teachers. Sex education is no exception. Mothers have told me over and over again, "We need help."[1]

American society has a tremendous stake in the success of sex education, for the negative consequences of ignorance, denial, and miscalculation ripple out well beyond the individual. We all share in the short-term economic costs of unemployment, welfare dependency, and medical costs that come with high rates of teen pregnancy, STDs, and HIV. We all share the long-term costs as well that come with inadequate parenting and lack of community support for teen parents and their children, with the result that many adults are unable to act responsibly or independently. For young people to understand that private lives exist in a public context and that we all have public as well as private responsibilities, schools, community agencies, religious institutions, the media, businesses, health care providers, and government at all levels need to become more involved in sex education. But punitive or directive measures alone are not enough; our gestures need to be caring, creative, and interactive to register fully with teens. If we can provide our girls with multiple resources and people beyond the family who care about them, I believe we can encourage more thoughtful decision-making and behavior.

Just as I have advocated ending the legacy of silence about sex in our home, I call on community leaders across America, with all their divergent opinions, to end the legacy of silence in society. Teens need conversations about sexuality in its largest context at school, doctors' offices, clubs, and places of worship, so that they can acquire the right facts to care for themselves, the skills to think for themselves, and the confidence and good judgment to make their own decisions. So much of what now happens under the umbrella of "sex education" fails to have an impact on teens. How much more effective we could be if we turned our collective attention to engaging all the relevant resources of the community.

## Improving the Health Care Connection

Experts in adolescent medicine would give Estelle Brown and Emily Shattuck high marks for ensuring that their daughters had a comfortable relationship with a physician who was interested in helping girls address both the physical and emotional aspects of sex. I wish we could provide this for all girls. Unfortunately, two major obstacles stand in the way. First, more than four out of ten teenagers have no health insurance. (Even among those who do have insurance, some teens do not take advantage of it because they are concerned about issues of confidentiality or they view health care as not important.) Second, many physicians are reluctant or unprepared to talk with teens about sexual matters, and they often hesitate to ask questions about sexual activity and contraceptive use.[2]

Physicians' hesitancy and unpreparedness have plagued adolescent health care for a number of years. As long ago as 1978 the American Academy of Pediatrics recommended changes in the medical school curriculum that would better prepare pediatricians to provide adolescent health care. At the time these recommendations were made, 66 percent of pediatricians judged themselves insufficiently trained in adolescent medicine. In 1989, when 3,000 pediatricians were asked to assess their training in adolescent medicine, 55 percent still considered it insufficient. And as recently as 1994, when residents in urban hospitals who were most likely to interact with teenagers evaluated their preparation to deal with adolescent health issues, they "did not feel well-prepared for topics relating to sexuality, endocrinology, contraception, or psychosocial problems. Pediatricians in particular were hesitant about gynecology, especially pregnancy and contraception."[3]

Compounding the insufficiency of medical training is the fact that teen life doesn't lend itself easily to adolescent sexual health care. A medical school pediatrician, when asked how we might provide more consistent health care for adolescents, reminded me that teenagers don't carry appointment books and rarely seek out doctors. "We see them when they are really sick, when they need an exam for sports or camp or shots for travel." Even when a teen does visit a primary care physician or gynecologist, if she has one, it is unlikely that the subject of sex will be raised by the physician. For example, of approximately 2,000 ninth- through twelfth-grade students in an urban Los Angeles school district, only a small percentage had discussed a sex-related topic with a doctor. A mere 15 percent had talked about their sexual activity, and only 13 percent about how to say no to unwanted sex. One of the most frequently raised topics was AIDS, with 39 percent discussing it with their doctor. In another study of adolescents consulting health care providers, "while 70% said they wanted to address STDs with their doctors, and 66% wanted to address contraception, these topics were actually discussed only 18% and 22% of the time respectively." Half the females in the study felt the practitioner should start the conversation because teenagers were too shy to do so themselves.[4]

The message seems clear: many teenage girls would welcome a conversation with a trusted health care provider, but most will not begin the conversation, and many practitioners are not trained to feel competent or comfortable discussing these issues. As one pediatrician noted, doctors feel that adolescents are not interested or are uncomfortable or distrustful when it comes to talking about sex.[5]

Both teenagers and our communities stand to benefit if residents in pediatrics, family medicine, ob-gyn, and internal medicine received focused training in adolescent medicine. And perhaps, if consumers demand it, the health industry will make more concerted efforts to encourage training in this field. Planned Parenthood advises that a girl begin seeing a gynecologist when she is eighteen or when she becomes sexually active, whichever comes first; if all teens followed this advice, it would be all the more important to have adequately trained health care providers in place.[6]

Economics will always play a role in access to health care, but for those girls who lack health insurance, there are, thankfully, federally funded clinics that offer contraceptive care, among other health benefits. For girls under eighteen, that care must be provided free of charge and parental notification is not necessary.[7]

Another important connection that is currently missing is good communication between schools and health care providers. For health care to be truly "accessible" to teens, it should be at school or nearby, where adolescents are apt to be and feel comfortable. More school-based and school-linked clinics could provide better accessibility and, in some cases, free services to adolescents who might not otherwise seek care. Approximately three hundred such school-based clinics are in place now, but they serve only a fraction of the teen population, and providing contraception is often verboten.[8]

Health services for teens can also be based in health maintenance organizations (HMOs), private physicians' offices, or neighborhood clinics. For the community of Jefferson High, medical and social services staff at the school and the neighborhood health center communicated frequently about the needs of individual students. When they realized they were dealing with many of the same issues, particularly with regard to high-risk behaviors of teens, they collaborated on applying for a grant for federal funding to provide additional support staff at the school. The Jefferson model is one that other schools and community health care providers could aspire to. Since these two groups are often dealing with the same subset of adolescents in a particular community, it makes sense for them to work together on teen health care.

## Improving Sex Education in Our Schools

Comprehensive sex education can help teenagers delay intercourse, and, if they do engage in intercourse, can promote the use of contraception to prevent pregnancy and STDs. That's the good news. The discouraging news is that much sex education in American schools today falls dreadfully short of being comprehensive. In particular, abstinence-*only* education, to which a small percentage of schools subscribes, has failed to achieve the stated goals of those who advocate it. Granted, teens in some of these programs have shown increases in knowledge about sexuality and shifts in attitudes about sexual decision-making, but no statistically significant evidence supports the claim that abstinence-only programs are effective in delaying sexual intercourse among adolescents.[9]

If we define "success" in sex education as reducing sexual risk-taking behavior among teens, those programs that do succeed typically are characterized by a narrow focus on that goal. Such programs work on reducing behaviors that may lead to HIV-STD infection or unintended pregnancy. The curriculum provides basic, accurate information about the risks of unprotected intercourse and the methods of avoiding it; recognizes social influences, changing individual values, and media influences; reinforces individual beliefs and group norms against unprotected sex; and includes a variety of communication strategies, including peer counseling and negotiation and refusal skills.[10]

Although comprehensive sexuality programs have been disappointing in their effectiveness — partly because our expectations were unrealistically high and partly because program evaluations have not been designed to measure small effects — there is room for optimism. Both programs and evaluations are improving, and there is now evidence that a few programs that are abstinence-based but provide contraceptive information and/or referral services have reduced unprotected intercourse among teens, either by delaying the initiation of intercourse or by increasing the use of condoms and other contraceptives.[11]

The well-meaning folks who argue vehemently in community forums and school board meetings that we ought not to tell girls like Angela, Carmen, and Carolyn what we know about contraception, HIV, pregnancy, and sexuality speak with the fierce conviction that talking about sex is dangerous for teens. "Don't give them the choice,

and they won't make the mistake" is how one public advocate of abstinence-only education explained his views.[12] When those speaking out
against comprehensive sex education talk about keeping teens safe
and healthy, few disagree with that goal. No mainstream group in
America interested in sex education — not Planned Parenthood, not
the Sexuality Information and Education Council of the United States
(SIECUS), not the Alan Guttmacher Institute, to name three of the
most recognized groups — wants to encourage adolescent sexual activity. All of us are concerned with our teens' safety and well-being; it is
how to ensure this result that stirs up contention.

On its face, abstinence-*based* education may look similar to
abstinence-*only* education, but the two are quite different. A California report on school sex education curriculums explains the two approaches this way: "Most comprehensive sex education curricula are
abstinence-based. Their underlying goal is to encourage students to be
responsible for and knowledgeable about their own health, coming
from the notion that sexual activity can have negative outcomes on
young people. These programs help students acquire skills to say no to
unwanted sexual activity and encourage them to postpone sex until
they are truly ready for it." Such an approach, the report continues,
provides "students with a full range of information about sexual health,
including information about contraception and safer sex precautions
for those students who are already sexually active and for those who
will be at some point in their future."[13] The majority of mainstream sex
educators support abstinence-based comprehensive sex education.

By contrast, for abstinence-only school programs in California, the
same report concludes that "these curricula deny students information
about contraception practices to avoid the transmission of HIV and
other sexually transmitted diseases and other sexual health issues."
One expert characterized the programs as "fear based," relying on fear
and shame to discourage students from engaging in sexual behavior,
and said that they "typically omit critical information, contain medical
mis-information, include sexist and anti-choice bias and often have a
foundation in fundamentalist religious belief." Whatever their foundation, abstinence-only programs appear to work at cross-purposes with

what we know about teens. If approximately 60 percent of teens have sex by age eighteen, is it logical to avoid that reality in our school education? Do we honestly believe that 60 percent will stop having sex if we don't talk about contraception? There is no reliable evidence to suggest that providing information about contraception leads to an increase in sexual activity; quite the contrary, the impact of comprehensive sex education programs seems most significant with those adolescents who are already or are preparing to become sexually active.[14]

It stands to reason that the strongest, most curious, most intellectually restless adolescents will be the very ones who most resent and resist fear-based, shame-oriented tactics. There is something challenging and provocative in being told we can't be told, in being lectured to in ways that don't square with our own perceptions and feelings. How many of us have asked a teen not to do something and seen her purposefully engage in the prohibited behavior? Adolescence is a time of challenging and testing out. Not acknowledging that in our teaching methods seems a precarious and ill-advised approach.

The content of our adolescents' sexuality education depends heavily on the community they live in. Because the federal government is precluded from setting state and local curriculum standards, each state formulates its own guidelines, and local schools shape their programs accordingly. Most of the states either recommend or require some form of sex education. Too often, however, the curriculums are weakened by compromise. In 1995 twenty-two states and the District of Columbia required schools to provide both sexuality and STD/HIV education, but *thirteen states lacked any requirements related to sexuality education.* While twenty-six states insisted that the curriculum include abstinence instruction, only fourteen of them also stipulated that information be provided on contraception, pregnancy, and disease prevention.[15]

Some states have taken the initiative to teach students that sex does not happen in a vacuum, that there are a host of issues to consider. In 1995 more than half of the states mandated that schools provide family life education, including information on dating and interpersonal relationships. About the same proportion required or recommended instruc-

tion on decision-making skills, such as resisting peer pressure and setting limits during dates. This is an important backdrop for students' understanding of sex. Yet mandates can also work to stop conversation:
eight states required or recommended teaching that homosexuality is
not an acceptable lifestyle and/or that homosexual conduct is a criminal
offense under state law. Five states prohibited discussion of abortion.[16]

Although we have ample evidence to support the conclusion that
abstinence-only education is ineffective with teens, the federal government appears to be intent on ignoring what works for adolescents.
Most recently, in the final negotiations to pass the 1996 welfare law,
legislators appropriated $250 million over the next five years for absti-
nence-only education. It also proposed to shower a total of $400 mil-
lion on states that show no increase or that reduce the rate of teen
births outside of marriage, with no increase in abortions, over a two-
year period.

One is left to wonder why people who are not experts themselves
and who seem to ignore the findings of experts in adolescent development are shaping policy on such critical matters. It is hard to believe
that if they had looked at the evidence, policymakers would have created legislation that states as "its exclusive purpose" the "teaching [of]
the social, psychological, and health gains to be realized by abstaining
from sexuality activity." One of the more outrageous stipulations of
this legislation is that any class funded with federal monies should
teach "that sexual activity outside of the context of marriage is likely to
have harmful psychological and physical effects." This curriculum is
supposed to teach that "a mutually faithful monogamous relationship
in the context of marriage is the expected standard of human sexual
activity." Whose standard? These messages could be extremely harmful to teens who are already sexually active.

This new restriction on the use of federal funds has presented a
dilemma for many states and local communities. With community organizations and schools in desperate need of funds to implement and
sustain sexuality education programs, many feel they have been placed
in a no-win situation. If they apply for federal grants, they must exclude or deny what they know is important information for the sexual

health of youngsters. As one critic said, "abstinence-only programs do not allow [us] to respond honestly to young people's questions." Some educators have been trying to find ways to compete for these grants without compromising what they know to be the best methods for teaching sexual health to adolescents. Other states have resolved the dilemma by allocating the federal funds only to sex education classes for children fourteen and under.[17]

At the local level, however, some secondary schools have decided not to apply for the funds at all because they cannot in good conscience develop programs that will not only be unsuccessful but will present misleading and dishonest information. As one critic put it, "Congress may as well take $250 million . . . and put it through a shredder and feed it to cattle as give it to schools to teach abstinence to high school students."[18] The persistent misguided belief that comprehensive sexuality education will entice adolescents into having sex abandons our teens. We continue to give them no alternative to sexual abstinence.

The majority of people in this country want a more comprehensive approach to sexuality education, but they have abdicated any role in advocating for it. As the vocal minority has become more organized and diligent in lobbying for abstinence-only programs, the majority has remained mostly quiet and inactive. Unless those of us who understand the importance of comprehensive sexuality education become more involved in our communities and in lobbying our legislators, our adolescents will continue to be without the full spectrum of information they deserve.

## Something to Say Yes To

We have grown very adept at telling our teens when and what to say no to. We seem to have more trouble providing opportunities for adolescents to say yes. Edith Phelps, in her book *No Turning Back*, wisely writes, "As teenagers, girls are closely watching the scenarios of their own lives, even as they live them. They are wise enough to know that they must find their own way through the hazards of adolescence, but they must also have a right to the knowledge, skills and strategies that will steer them through the conflicting messages about their sexuality and their roles as women."[19] Where can girls find the knowledge and skills Phelps speaks of? They are looking to us, their mothers, sisters, aunts, and grandmothers; their teachers and advisers; their youth group leaders, coaches, and ministers; their mentors and heroines to see how we balance caring and coping; how we balance our own needs and those of other people in our lives; how we balance the personal and the professional.

Is this sex education? Of course it is. Deciding when and with whom we fall in love, when we hand over our hearts and then our bodies to someone else, when and how and where and with whom we will live — these decisions involve not just our sexuality but every aspect of our lives. We want girls to think about the challenging questions that their sexual awakening presents in the context of their whole lives: Why say no? What requirements must be fulfilled before they say yes? What markers of maturity, what accomplishments, come before yes? How girls learn to say yes — yes to their intellectual capabilities, to their athletic capabilities, and ultimately to their sexuality is all a part of sex education.

With support at home and opportunities through the community, girls can develop a firm sense of self-worth. Whether it's the Girl Scouts, Boys and Girls Club, Girls, Inc., the YWCA, church groups, sports teams, or other youth groups, group activities encourage girls' interests beyond the narrow scope of drugs, drinking, and sex. But they also provide a stage for peer dialogue and mentoring support, a place where girls can speak with others about their lives, their frustrations, and their values. Government should help provide funding for some of these programs, but it is at the local level that such grassroots opportunities come to life.

We know that girls who do well in school, sports, or other extracurricular activities often feel better about themselves, as happened with Carolyn Valentia. Strong self-esteem, we also know, contributes to more carefully considered decisions about initiating — or not initiating — sexual intercourse.[20] Adolescents who become involved in sports or music, for instance, and who have adults outside the family to talk with are also less likely to engage in a wide range of risky behaviors.

Because adolescents cannot vote, they are a constituency without a political voice and without much leverage. Therefore it falls to parents to help politicians appreciate the importance of funding not only improved health opportunities and comprehensive and informed sexuality programs but also a whole range of community youth programs.

Let us all — mothers, fathers, community leaders, ministers, policymakers, and countless others involved in the lives of adolescents — encourage our girls to embrace life. As they become young women — stretching, experimenting, but always learning — we can help them feel comfortable with their bodies and with their decisions by providing a sounding board, offering our thoughts and feelings, and giving them affirmation. Raising knowledgeable, informed, and confident daughters is an important job. Adding sexuality to the conversation, I passionately believe, will help them to feel comfortable with their sexuality, to enjoy the pleasures and rights of young womanhood, using their good sense.

As mothers today, we have benefited from changing values and unprecedented opportunities for women. Now we have the chance to be a major influence in our girls' lives. We can give them a new legacy of respect and self-esteem by teaching them about sex and sexuality in new ways. It is our privilege, our right, and our powerful responsibility to do so.

**APPENDIX**

**NOTES**

**BIBLIOGRAPHY**

**INDEX**

# Organizations

ALAN GUTTMACHER INSTITUTE
120 Wall Street
New York, NY 10005
212-248-1111
Fax: 212-248-1951
Email/Web page: www.agi-usa.org

AMERICAN ACADEMY
OF PEDIATRICS
National Headquarters:
141 Northwest Point Boulevard
Elk Grove Village, IL 60007-1098
847-228-5005
Fax: 847-228-5097
Email/Web page: www.aap.org

AMERICAN ASSOCIATION OF
UNIVERSITY WOMEN
1111 16th Street NW
Washington, DC 20036
202-785-7700
Fax: 202-872-1425
TDD: 202-785-7777
Email: info@mail.aauw.org
Web page: www.aauw.org

THE AMERICAN COLLEGE
OF OBSTETRICIANS AND
GYNECOLOGISTS
409 12th Street SW
Washington, DC 20024-2188
202-638-5577
Fax: 202-484-5107

ETR ASSOCIATES
PO Box 1830
Santa Cruz, CA 95061-1830
800-321-4407

GIRL POWER!
Department of Health and Human
    Services
National Clearinghouse for Alcohol
    and Drug Information (NCADI)
800-729-6686 (TDD 1-800-487-4889)
Web page: www.health.org/gpower

GIRLS, INC
Resource Center
441 West Michigan Street
Indianapolis, IN 46202-3233
800-374-4475

GIRL SCOUTS OF THE
UNITED STATES
420 Fifth Avenue
New York, NY 10018-2798
800-221-6707 (for catalogue)
Email/Web page: www.gsusa.org

NATIONAL ABORTION RIGHTS
ACTION LEAGUE (NARAL)
1156 15th Street NW, Suite 700
Washington, DC 20005
Email/Web page: www.naral.org

NATIONAL ASSOCIATION FOR
GIRLS AND WOMEN IN SPORTS
1900 Association Drive
Reston, VA 20191
703-476-3450
Email: NAGWS@AAHPERD.ORG

NATIONAL CAMPAIGN TO
PREVENT TEEN PREGNANCY
Sarah S. Brown, Director
2100 M Street NW
Suite 300
Washington, DC 20037
202-857-8655
Fax: 202-331-7735
Email/Web page:
   www.teenpregnancy.org

NATIONAL ORGANIZATION ON
ADOLESCENT PREGNANCY,
PARENTING AND PREVENTION
1319 F Street NW, Suite 400
Washington, DC 20004
888-766-2777
Fax: 202-783-5775
Email: NOAPPP@EROLS.COM

PARENTS AND FRIENDS OF
LESBIANS AND GAYS (PFLAG)
1101 14th Street NW, Suite 1030
Washington DC 20005
202-638-4200
Fax: 202-638-0243
Email/Web page:
   INFO@PFLAG.ORG

PLANNED PARENTHOOD
FEDERATION OF AMERICA
810 Seventh Avenue
New York, NY 10019
800-669-0156
Fax: 212-261-4352
Email/Web page: www.ppfa.org

SEARCH INSTITUTE
Thresher Square West
700 S. 3rd Street
Suite 210
Minneapolis, MN 55415
612-376-8955
Fax: 612-376-8956
Web page: www.searchinstitute.org

SEXUALITY AND INFORMATION
COUNCIL OF THE UNITED
STATES (SIECUS)
Publications Department
130 West 42nd Street, Suite 350
New York, NY 10036-7802
212-819-9770
Fax: 212-819-9776
Email/Web page: www.siecus.org

SOCIETY FOR ADOLESCENT
MEDICINE
1916 Copper Oaks Circle
Blue Springs, MO 64015
816-224-8010
Fax: 816-224-8009
Email: SOCADMED@GVI.NET

WOMEN'S SPORTS FOUNDATION
Eisenhower Park, East Meadow
New York, NY 11554
800-227-3988
516-542-4700
Email/Web page: wosport@aol.com;
   www.lifetimetv.com/wosport

YWCA OF THE U.S.A.
Empire State Building
Suite 301
350 Fifth Avenue
New York, NY 10118
212-273-7800
Fax: 212-465-2281
Email/Web page: www.ywca.org

# Notes

1. IT'S ABOUT TIME: NEW TIMES, NEW TALK

1. On teen pregnancy rates, see "Adolescent Pregnancy Fact Sheet" (Washington, D.C.: American College of Obstetrics and Gynecology, 1996). On teens' knowledge of sexually transmitted diseases, see *STD News: A Quarterly Newsletter of the American Social Health Association* 3, no. 2 (Winter 1996): 1–5.

2. See Mary Pipher, *Reviving Ophelia: Saving the Selves of Adolescent Girls* (New York: Ballantine Books, 1994), pp. 203–18, 244, 245.

3. Maternity Care Coalition of Philadelphia, "Teen Discussion Group Summary Report," June 1996.

4. The survey is discussed in Michael D. Resnick et al., "Protecting Adolescents from Harm: Findings from the National Longitudinal Study on Adolescent Health," *Journal of the American Medical Association* 278, no. 10 (Sept. 10, 1997): 823–32.

5. On the importance of family and the primacy of mother-daughter relationships, see Nancy Chodorow, *The Reproduction of Mothering: Psychoanalysis and the Sociology of Gender* (Berkeley: University of California Press, 1978); Susan F. Newcomer and J. Richard Udry, "Mothers' Influence on the Sexual Behavior of Their Teenage Children," *Journal of Marriage and the Family*, May 1984, pp. 477–85; Judith K. Inazu and Greer Litton Fox, "Maternal Influence on the Sexual Behavior of Teenage Daughters," *Journal of Family Issues* 1, no. 1 (1980): 81–101; Jeanne Brooks-Gunn and Frank F. Furstenberg, "Adolescent Sexual Behavior," *American Psychologist* 44 (1989): 249–57; Douglas Kirby et al., "School-Based Programs to Reduce Sexual Risk Behaviors: A Review of Effectiveness," *Public Health Reports* 109, no. 3 (May/June 1994) and James Jaccard, Patricia J. Dittus, and Vivian V. Gordon, "Maternal Correlates of Adolescent Sexual and Contraceptive Behavior," *Family Planning Perspectives* 28, no. 4 (July/August 1996): 159–85.

6. U.S. Department of Health and Human Services, Center for Disease Control and Prevention, National Center for Health Statistics, *Vital and Health Statistics: Fertility, Family Planning, and Women's Health: New Data from the 1995 National Survey on Family Growth*, series 23, no. 19 (May 1947), 30. Kristin A. Moore, *Facts at a Glance* (Washington, D.C.: Child Trends, 1996); Sarah S. Brown and Leon Eisenberg, *The Best Intentions: Unintended Pregnancy and the*

*Well-Being of Children and Families* (Washington, D.C.: National Academy Press, 1995), p. 96; and Carnegie Council on Adolescent Development, *Great Transitions: Preparing Adolescents for a New Century* (New York: Carnegie Corporation, 1995), p. 24.

7. See "State-Specific Pregnancy and Birth Rates among Teenagers — U.S. 1991–1992," *Morbidity and Mortality Week in Review* 44, no. 37 (Sept. 22, 1995): 677–700; Alison M. Spitz et al., "Pregnancy, Abortion and Birth Rates among US Adolescents — 1980, 1985 and 1990," *Journal of the American Medical Association* 275, no. 13 (April 3, 1996): 989–94; Brown and Eisenberg, *Best Intentions*, pp. 94–95.

8. See Carol Gilligan, *In a Different Voice: Psychological Theory and Women's Development* (Cambridge: Harvard University Press, 1982).

9. Carnegie Council, *Great Transitions*, pp. 10, 42.

10. Joan S. Coombs, "Society Must Take Some Responsibility," *Philadelphia Inquirer*, December 8, 1996.

## 2. PARALLEL WORLDS: THE GIRLS OF
## JEFFERSON AND NOTTINGHAM HIGH SCHOOLS

1. The questionnaire, which was adapted from H. L. Barnes and D. H. Olson, "Parent-Adolescent Communication," is available from Family Social Science, University of Minnesota, 290 McNeal Hall, St. Paul, Minn. 55108.

2. For more on African-American mothers and daughters, see P. H. Collins, "The Meaning of Motherhood in Black Culture and Black Mother-Daughter Relationships," *Sage: A Scholarly Journal on Black Women* 4, no. 2 (1987): 3–10; Consortium for Research on Black Adolescence, *Black Adolescence: Current Issues and Annotated Bibliography* (Boston: G. K. Hall, 1990); and G. Joseph, "Mothers and Daughters: Traditional and New Perspectives, *Sage* 1, no. 2 (1984): 17–21.

## 3. FROM LITTLE GIRL TO YOUNG VENUS:
## NURTURING GIRLS THROUGH ADOLESCENCE

1. American Association of University Women, *Shortchanging Girls, Shortchanging America: A Call to Action* (Washington, D.C.: American Association of University Women, 1991). Carol Gilligan, "In a Different Voice: Women's Conceptions of the Self and of Morality," *Harvard Educational Review* 47 (1977).

2. Erik Erikson, *Identity, Youth and Crisis* (New York: W. W. Norton, 1968).

3. Erik Erikson, *Childhood and Society*, 2nd ed. (New York: W. W. Norton, 1963), pp. 261, 263.

4. See, for example, Sigmund Freud, "Three Essays on the Theory of Sexuality," in James Strachey, ed. and trans., *The Complete Psychological Works of Sigmund Freud*, vol. 7 (London: Hogarth Press, 1905); and Barbel Inhelder and Jean Piaget, *The Growth of Logical Thinking from Childhood to Adolescence* (New York: Basic Books, 1958).

5. See Chodorow, *Reproduction of Mothering*; Gilligan, *In a Different Voice*; Jean Baker Miller, *Toward a New Psychology of Women* (Boston: Beacon Press, 1976; rev. ed., 1982).

6. Lynn M. Brown and Carol Gilligan, *Meeting at the Crossroads* (New York: Ballantine Books, 1992).

7. See Julius B. Richmond, "Human Development," in *The Health of Americans, The American Assembly*, ed. B. Jones (Englewood Cliffs, N.J.: Prentice-Hall, 1990), pp. 5–37; and Roberta G. Simmons and Dale A. Blyth, *Moving into Adolescence: The Impact of Pubertal Change and School Context* (Hawthorne, N.Y.: Aldine De Gruyter, 1987).

8. See Fox and Inazu, "Patterns and Outcomes of Mother-Daughter Communication"; and Eileen Hepburn, "A Three-Level Model of Parent-Daughter Communication about Sexual Topics," *Adolescence* 18, no. 71 (1983): 523–34.

9. See Terri Apter, *Altered Loves: Mothers and Daughters during Adolescence* (New York: St. Martin's Press, 1990); and Gilligan, *In a Different Voice*.

10. See Deborah L. Tolman and Tracy E. Higgins, "How Being a Good Girl Can Be Bad for Girls," In *Bad Girls, Good Girls: Women, Sex and Power in the Nineties*, ed. Nan Bauer Maglin and Donna Perry (New Brunswick, N.J.: Rutgers University Press, 1996), pp. 205–25.

11. Apter, *Altered Loves*, p. 219.

12. See Pipher, *Reviving Ophelia*, pp. 101–14.

## 4. NUTS AND BOLTS AND MORE:
## WHAT ADOLESCENT GIRLS KNOW ABOUT SEX

1. Seth D. Ammerman et al., "Do Adolescents Understand What Physicians Say about Sexuality and Health?" *Clinical Pediatrics* (October 1992): 590–95.

2. Marilyn Hockenberry-Eaton et al., "Mother and Adolescent Knowledge of Sexual Development: The Effect of Gender, Age and Sexual Experience," *Adolescence* 31, no. 121 (Spring 1996): 35–47

3. On teens' misconceptions about sex, see Maternity Care Coalition, "Teen Discussion Group Summary Report"; Ammerman et al., "Do Adolescents Understand What Physicians Say"; and "Teen Sex and Pregnancy" fact sheet (New York: Alan Guttmacher Institute, June 1997; available through the Internet at http://www.agi usa.org/pubs/fb_teensex1.html#4a).

4. On definitions of puberty, see *Adolescent Health*, vol. 1: *Summary and Policy Options* (Washington, D.C.: U.S. Congress, Office of Technology Assessment, April 1991).

5. Marcia E. Herman-Giddens et al., "Secondary Sexual Characteristics and Menses in Young Girls Seen in Office Practice: A Study from the Pediatric Research in Office Settings Network," *Pediatrics* 99, no. 4 (April 1997): 505–12.

6. Brenda C. Coleman, "Study Finds Earlier Onset of Puberty for American Girls," *Philadelphia Inquirer*, April 8, 1997, p. A7.

7. See Richmond, "Human Development," pp. 5–37; and Simmons and Blyth, *Moving into Adolescence*.

8. For more on instructing girls about menstruation, see Margaret L. Stubbs, Jill Rierdan, and Elissa Koff, *Becoming a Woman: Considerations in Educating Adolescents about Menstruation*, Working Paper 169, rev. version (Wellesley, Mass.: Wellesley College Center for Research on Women, 1988); Elissa Koff and Jill Rierdan, "Preparing Girls for Menstruation: Recommendations from Adolescent Girls," *Adolescence* 30, no. 120 (Winter 1995): 795–811; and Elissa Koff and Jill Rierdan, "Early Adolescent Girls' Understanding of Menstruation," *Women and Health* 22, no. 4 (1995): 1–19.

9. Stubbs, Rierdan, and Koff, *Becoming a Woman*.

10. *Runner's World* did a story on this event (John Brant, "Cosmas Stumbles, Uta Rumbles," *Runner's World*, July 1996, p. 50). According to Cristina Negron, senior editor of the magazine (personal communication, December 1, 1997), Pippig's finish was "nothing but heroic." She does not recall that coverage of Pippig was mixed but rather that it was lauded as heroic. She acknowledges that members of the general public may have found the episode distasteful.

11. On teenage pregnancy rates, see Kristin Luker, *Dubious Conceptions: The Politics of Teenage Pregnancy* (Cambridge: Harvard University Press, 1996); Brown and Eisenberg, *Best Intentions*; and *National Campaign to Prevent Teen Pregnancy Newsletter* (Washington, D.C., Summer 1997).

12. Caitlin Ryan and Dona Futterman, "Overview: HIV Infection in Adolescents Including Lesbian and Gay Males," in *Lesbian and Gay Youth: Care and Counseling. Adolescent Medicine: State of the Art Reviews* 8, no. 2 (June 1997): 309–14.

13. See Douglas Kirby et al., "School-Based Programs to Reduce Sexual Risk Behaviors: A Review of Effectiveness," *Public Health Reports* 109, no. 3 (May/June 1994): 339–59; Phyllida Burlingame, *Sex, Lies and Politics: Abstinence-Only Curricula in California Public Schools* (Oakland, Calif.: Applied Research Center, May 1997).

14. On the prevalence of STDs, see Thomas R. Eng and William T. Butler, eds., *The Hidden Epidemic: Confronting Sexually Transmitted Diseases* (Washington, D.C.: National Academy Press, 1996); Paula K. Braverman and Victor C. Strasburger, "Sexually Transmitted Diseases," *Clinical Pediatrics* (January 1994): 26–37; and *Sexually Transmitted Diseases in the United States* (New York: Sexuality Information and Education Council of the United States, 1997; available through the Internet at http://www.siecus.org/pubs/fact/fact0008.html). On chlamydia, see Braverman and Strasburger, "Sexually Transmitted Diseases." On gonorrhea, see C. Wayne Sells and Robert W. Blum, "Morbidity and Mortality among US Adolescents: An Overview of Data and Trends," *American Journal of Public Health* 86, no. 4 (April 1961): 513–19. On STD rates, see "Fact Sheet: Sexually Transmitted Diseases (STDs) in the United States: Exposing the Epidemic" (New York: Alan Guttmacher Institute, Henry J. Kaiser Family Foundation, and National Press Foundation, November 20, 1996).

15. *STD News* 3, no. 2: 1, 5.

16. Tamar Lewin: "Fearing Disease, Teens Alter Sexual Practices," *New York Times*, April 5, 1997, National Report section; see also Mark A. Schuster, Robert M. Bell, and David E. Kanouse, "The Sexual Practices of Adolescent Virgins: Genital Sexual Activities of High School Graduate Students Who Have Never Had Sexual Intercourse," *American Journal of Public Health* 86, no. 11 (November 1996): 1570–76.

17. Lewin, "Fearing Disease."

18. Ibid.

19. See Robert A. Hatcher et al., *Contraceptive Technology: 1990–1992*, 15th rev. ed. (New York: Irvington, 1990); Brown and Eisenberg, *Best Intentions*.

20. Maternity Care Coalition, "Teen Discussion Group Summary Report," June 1996.

21. On issues around the use of birth control pills, see U.S. Department of Health and Human Services, *Fertility, Family Planning and Women's Health,* p. 49. On rationalizations for not using contraception, see Greer Litton Fox and Judith K. Inazu, "Patterns and Outcomes of Mother-Daughter Communication about Sexuality," *Journal of Social Issues* 36, no. 1 (1980): 7–29; and Sharon Thompson, "Putting a Big Thing into a Little Hole: Teenage Girls' Accounts of Sexual Initiation," *Journal of Sex Research* 27, no. 1 (February 1990): 81–94.

22. See Kirby et al., "School-Based Programs."

23. Parental consent requirements: National Abortion Rights Action League, July 1997.

24. See "Teenagers, Abortion, and Government Intrusion Laws" (New York: Planned Parenthood Federation of America, 1997; available through the Internet at http://www.ppfa.org/ppfa/ab-teens.html).

25. On the feelings of lesbian teenagers, see Lauren Hartman, *Solutions: The Woman's Crisis Handbook* (Boston: Houghton Mifflin, 1997), pp. 82–88; Laura S. Kastner and Jennifer F. Wyatt, *The Seven-Year Stretch: How Families Work Together to Grow Through Adolescence* (Boston: Houghton Mifflin, 1997); Mary J. Rotheram-Borus and M. Isabela Fernandez, "Sexual Orientation and Developmental Challenges Experienced by Gay and Lesbian Youths," *Suicide and Life-Threatening Behavior* 25, suppl. (1995): 26–39; Ann Heron, ed., *Two Teenagers in Twenty: Writings by Gay and Lesbian Youth* (Los Angeles: Alyson Publications, 1983; rev. ed., Ann Heron, 1994); and Louise Rafkin, ed., *Different Daughters: A Book by Mothers of Lesbians,* 2nd ed. (Pittsburgh: Cleis Press, 1996).

## 5. BEYOND *BEVERLY HILLS 90210*: WHERE GIRLS GET THEIR INFORMATION

1. See Fox and Inazu, "Patterns and Outcomes of Mother-Daughter Communication," p. 11; Hepburn, "Three-Level Model," p. 527; Robert Coles and Geoffrey Stokes, *Sex and the American Teenager* (New York: Harper and Row, 1985), p. 96; J. Youniss and R. D. Ketterlinus, "Communication and Connectedness in Mother- and Father-Adolescent Relationships," *Journal of Youth and Adolescence* 16 (1987): 276; Apter, *Altered Loves,* pp. 124–57.

2. See Chodorow, *Reproduction of Mothering*; Sharon Rich, "Daughters View Their Relationships with Their Mothers," in *Making Connections: The Relational World of Adolescent Girls at Emma Willard School,* ed. Carol Gilligan, Naomi P. Lyons, and Trudy J. Hanmer (Cambridge, Mass.: Harvard University Press, 1990); and Fox and Inazu, "Patterns and Outcomes of Mother-Daughter Communication," p. 9.

3. Maternity Care Coalition, "Teen Discussion Group Summary Report."

4. Coles and Stokes, *Sex and the American Teenager,* p. 46.

5. *American Teens Speak: Sex, Myths, TV and Birth Control* (New York: Planned Parenthood Federation of America, 1986), as noted in Brent C. Miller and Greer Litton Fox, "Theories of Adolescent Heterosexual Behavior," *Journal of Adolescent Research* 2, no. 3 (1987): 269–82.

6. See Kaiser Family Foundation, *Sex, Kids and the Family Hour: A Three-Part Study of Sexual Content on Television* (Menlo Park, Calif.: Henry J. Kaiser Family Foundation, December 11, 1996; available through the Internet at http://www.

childrennow.org/media/FAMHOUR.html); S. Robert Lichter, Linda S. Lichter, and Stanley Rothman, *Prime Time: How TV Portrays American Culture* (Washington, D.C.: Regency Publishing, 1994), pp. 79–110; L. Monique Ward, "Talking about Sex: Common Themes about Sexuality in the Prime Time Television Programs Children and Adolescents View Most," *Journal of Youth and Adolescence* 24, no. 5 (1995), p. 605; Jane D. Brown and Jeanne R. Steele, *Sex and the Mass Media* (Menlo Park, Calif.: Henry J. Kaiser Family Foundation, 1995), pp. 1–9.

7. Ward, "Talking about Sex," p. 603.

8. On the prevalence of "worry-free sex," see Lichter, Lichter, and Rothman, *Prime Time*, p. 88. On the portrayal of sex as impersonal and exploitative, see Victor C. Strasburger, "Children, Adolescents and Television," *Pediatrics in Review* 13, no. 4 (1992): 144–51. On girls' fascination with media depiction of relationships, see Brown and Steele, *Sex and the Mass Media*, p. 9.

9. Ward, "Talking about Sex," p. 595; Brown and Steele, *Sex and the Mass Media*, p. 2; quote is from Strasburger, "Children, Adolescence and Television," p. 149.

10. Greenberg, B. S., J. D. Brown, and N. Buerkel-Rothfuss, *Media, Sex, and the Adolescent* (Creskill, N.J.: Hampton, 1993), p. 180, as cited in Victor C. Strasburger, *Adolescents and the Media: Medical and Psychological Impact* (Thousand Oaks, Calif.: Sage Publications, 1995), p. 45.

11. Elizabeth Debold, Marie Wilson, and Idelisse Malavé, *Mother-Daughter Revolution: From Betrayal to Power*, (New York: Addison-Wesley, 1993).

12. Ward, "Talking about Sex," p. 613; Brown and Steele, *Sex and the Mass Media*, p. 1; Maternity Care Coalition, "Teen Discussion Group Summary Report."

13. Kim Walsh Childers and Jane Brown, "Teen Media Awareness Mirrors Upbringing," *Media and Values* 46 (Spring 1989): 9.

14. Newton N. Minow and Craig L. Lamay, *Abandoned in the Wasteland: Children, Television and the First Amendment* (New York: Hill and Wang, 1995), p. 19.

15. Ward, "Talking about Sex," p. 609.

16. Lichter, Lichter, and Rothman, *Prime Time*, p. 88.

17. Maternity Care Coalition, "Teen Discussion Group Summary Report."

18. Brown and Steele, *Sex and the Mass Media*, p. 13.

19. Ibid., p 14.

20. *New York Times*, May 9, 1997, p. A13; *Philadelphia Inquirer*, April 20, 1997, pp. H1, H5.

21. Brown and Steele, *Sex and the Mass Media*, p. 13.

22. *The Kaiser Family Foundation Survey on Teens and Sex: What They Say Teens Need to Know and Who They Listen To* (Princeton, N.J.: Survey Research Associates, June 24, 1996).

23. Susan Ellis, Girls Incorporated (317–634–7546), personal communication. The Girls Incorporated Preventing Adolescent Pregnancy Program comprises "Growing Together: A Sexuality Education Program for Girls Ages 9–11," "Will Power/Won't Power: A Sexuality Education Program for Girls 12–14," "Taking Care of Business: A Sexuality and Career Exploration Program for Young Women Ages 15–18," and "Health Bridge: A Collaborative Model for Delivering Health Services to Young Women Ages 12–18," Girls Inc., National Resource Center, 441 W. Michigan Street, Indianapolis, IN 46202.

24. Information about the HHS Girl Power! campaign can be found through the Internet at http://www.health.org/gpower/media/forpress/hhscamp/html; http://www.health.org/gpower/campaign/linkend.html.

25. Michael McGee, vice president for education, Planned Parenthood of New York City (212–261–4627), personal communication.

26. Hartman, *Solutions*, p. 87.

## 6. WITH AN EYE TO THE FUTURE:
### DAUGHTER'S HOPES AND FEARS

1. See Catherine Stevens-Simon and Susan Reichert, "Sexual Abuse, Adolescent Pregnancy and Child Abuse: A Developmental Approach to an Intergenerational Cycle," *Archives of Pediatrics and Adolescent Medicine* 148, no. 1 (January 1994): 23–27.

2. Luker, *Dubious Conceptions*, pp. 136–38.

3. Lisbeth B. Schorr, *Within Our Reach: Breaking the Cycle of Disadvantage* (New York: Doubleday, 1988), p. 18; see also Luker, *Dubious Conceptions*, pp. 136–38.

4. On the risks to adolescent girls, see Pipher, *Reviving Ophelia*, p. 185; Carnegie Council, *Great Transitions*, pp. 24–25; Sells and Blum, "Morbidity and Mortality among US Adolescents," pp. 515–16; Lloyd D. Johnson, Patrick M. O'Malley, and Jerald G. Bachman, *National Survey Results on Drug Use from the Monitoring the Future Study, 1975–1994* (Rockville, Md.: U.S. Department of Health and Human Services, Public Health Service, National Institutes of Health, National Institute on Drug Use, 1995); Robert H. Durant et al., "Tobacco and Alcohol Use Behaviors Portrayed in Music Videos: A Content Analysis," *American Journal of Public Health* 87, no. 7 (July 1997): pp. 1131–135; U.S. General Accounting Office, *Welfare Dependency: Coordinated Efforts Can Better Serve Young At-Risk Teen Girls*, GAO/HEH/RCED-95-108 (Washington, D.C.: U.S. General Accounting Office, 1995); Sey Chassler, "What Teenage Girls Say about Pregnancy," *Parade*, February 2, 1997, p. 4; "Getting Ready or Not for Sex," *Boston Globe*, June 25, 1997, p. D6.

5. At the conclusion of my interview with Katrina, she and I talked about a checklist to help girls make a decision about sexual activity. Here are the ten questions that came out of our discussion.

1. Do I know what I should know about sex and have I thought it through?
2. Does being sexually active at this time in my life fit with my values and my family's values?
3. Do I really care about this person and does he care about me?
4. Have we developed a friendship?
5. Do I know how to protect myself from an unwanted pregnancy and/or AIDS and other sexually transmitted diseases?
6. Do I know where I can obtain contraceptives?
7. Have I talked over the use of contraceptives with my boyfriend and is it a mutual decision?
8. Do I know something about his previous sexual encounters?
9. Is this person someone I might want to be with for a long while and/or possibly marry in the future?

10. Do I think I am prepared to deal with any consequences that may result from this behavior?

6. David J. Landry and Jacqueline D. Forrest, "How Old Are U.S. Fathers?" *Family Planning Perspectives* 27, no. 4 (1995): 159–61, 165; Jennifer Steinhauer, "Study Cites Adult Males for the Most Teen-Age Births," *New York Times*, August 2, 1995, p. A10; Mike Males and Kenneth Chew, "The Age of Fathers in California Adolescent Births, 1993," *American Journal of Public Health* 84, no. 4 (April 1996): 565–68.

7. Katherine Seelye, "Concealing a Pregnancy to Avoid Telling Mom," *New York Times*, June 15, 1997, p. E5; "Sex and Consequences: Prom Case Should Prompt Questions about Society" (editorial), *Philadelphia Inquirer*, June 25, 1997, p. A–16; Amy Goodnough and Bruce Weber, "Before Prom Night, Suspect Was the Girl Next Door," *New York Times*, July 2, 1997, Metro Section.

8. See Eng and Butler, *Hidden Epidemic*; Mary Lou Lindegren et al., "Epidemiology of Human Immunodeficiency Virus Infection in Adolescents, United States," *Pediatric Infectious Diseases Journal* 13 (1994): 525–35; Alvin Goldfarb, "Adolescent Sexuality," in *Adolescent Gynecology and Endocrinology: Basic and Clinical Aspects*, ed. George Creatsas, George Mastorakos, and George P. Chrousos, Annals of the New York Academy of Science 816 (New York: New York Academy of Science, 1997).

9. Maternity Care Coalition, "Teen Discussion Group Summary Report."

## 7. WITH AN EYE TOWARD INDEPENDENCE: MOTHERS' HOPES AND FEARS

1. On the importance of physical attractiveness, see Nancy Friday, *The Power of Beauty* (New York: Harper Collins, 1996); and Grace Baruch, Rosalind Barnett, and Caryl Rivers, *Lifeprints: New Patterns of Love and Work for Today's Women* (New York: Signet Books, 1983), p. 252. Peggy Orenstein, *School Girls: Young Women, Self-Esteem and the Confidence Gap* (New York: Doubleday, 1994).

2. Pennsylvania Consolidated Statutes Annotated, Title 18, Sections 3121 and 3122.1.

3. Steinhauer, "Study Cites Adult Males," p. A10.

## 8. SPEAKING THE UNSPOKEN: SEXUAL DESIRE

1. Paula Webster, "The Forbidden Eroticism and Taboo," in Carol S. Vance, ed., *Pleasure and Danger: Exploring Female Sexuality* (Boston: Routledge and Kegan Paul, 1984), p. 385.

2. U.S. Department of Health and Human Services, *Fertility, Family Planning and Women's Health*, p. 30.

3. Susan K. Flinn and Susan A. Messina, "The Politics of Desire: The Touchy Subject of Success in Sex Education," *Bryn Mawr Alumnae Bulletin* (1996): 12–15.

4. Dalma Heyn, *The Erotic Silence of the American Wife* (New York: Random House, 1992), p. 70.

5. Tolman and Higgins, "How Being a Good Girl Can be Bad," p. 208.

6. Michelle Fine, "Sexuality, Schooling and Adolescent Females: The Missing Discourse of Desire," *Educational Review* 58 (1988): 33.

7. See Theresa Crenshaw, *The Alchemy of Love and Lust* (Putnam, 1996), pp. 15–16.

8. Carol Vance and Carol A. Pollis, "Introduction: A Special Issue on Feminist Perspectives and Sexuality," *Journal of Sex Research* 27, no. 1 (February 1990): 1–5; Fine, "Sexuality, Schooling and Adolescent Females," pp. 29–53; Michelle Fine and Nancie Zane, "Being Wrapped Too Tight: When Low-Income Women Drop Out of High School," in *Dropouts from School*, ed. L. Weis, R. Farrar, and H. Petire (New York: State University of New York Press, 1989), pp. 23–53; Tolman and Higgins, "How Being a Good Girl Can Be Bad," pp. 205–25; Deborah L. Tolman, "Discourses of Adolescent Girls' Sexual Desire in Developmental Psychology and Feminist Scholarship," qualifying paper, Harvard Graduate School of Education, 1990; Sharon Thompson, *Going All the Way: Teenage Girls' Tales of Sex, Romance and Pregnancy* (New York: Hill and Wang, 1995), pp. 341–61; Elizabeth Debold, Marie Wilson, and Idelisse Malavé, *Mother-Daughter Revolution: From Betrayal to Power* (New York: Addison-Wesley, 1993), pp. 169–95.

9. This survey is available through the Internet at http://www.compbio.caltech.edu/-dliney/pics/in_tray/synonyms.html.

10. In this sample, women with at least one adolescent daughter between the ages of ten and twenty were invited to complete a five-page open-ended questionnaire. The majority of these women had family incomes in the range of $25,000 to $100,000; 8 percent reported incomes under $25,000, and 8 percent over $200,000. All but one of the mothers had graduated from high school, and 27 percent held college degrees. Approximately one-fourth of the college graduates had master's degrees, and another 10 percent had done additional postbaccalaureate work. Sixty-two percent of the women were married; 27 percent were either divorced or separated. Fifty-three percent were Protestant, 20 percent Jewish, and 13 percent Catholic. Another 14 percent indicated no religious affiliation. The majority of respondents resided in Pennsylvania (48 percent) or Texas (41 percent); 6 percent lived in California.

11. One of the women had been raped when she was five; this was not factored into the average age of intercourse. The earliest age of initiation was eight; the latest, "late twenties." Fifty-two percent reported using contraception — pills, condoms, or both — when they first had intercourse, and 42 percent noted that no contraception had been used.

12. Debold, Wilson, and Malavé, *Mother-Daughter Revolution: From Betrayal to Power,* p. 169, p. 173.

13. Debold, Wilson, and Malavé, *Mother-Daughter Revolution: From Betrayal to Power,* pp. 189–191; Naomi Wolf, *Promiscuities: The Secret Struggle for Womanhood* (New York: Random House, 1997).

## 9. OUT OF THE LOOP: GETTING FATHERS INVOLVED

1. Apter, *Altered Loves*, p. 68.

2. See R. Montemayor, M. Eberly, and D. J. Flannery, "Effects of Pubertal Status and Conversation Topic on Parent and Adolescent Affective Expression," *Journal of Early Adolescence* 13 (1993): 431–47; and R. W. Larson, "Finding Time for Fatherhood: The Emotional Ecology of Adolescent-Father Interactions," in

S. Shulman and W. A. Collins, eds., *Father-Adolescent Relationships* (San Francisco: Jossey-Bass, 1993), pp. 7–25.

3. Goodman quoted in Victoria Secunda, *Women and Their Fathers: The Sexual and Romantic Impact of the First Man in Your Life* (New York: Delacorte Press, 1992), p. 98.

4. Linda Beth Tiedje and Cynthia Darling-Fisher, "Fatherhood Reconsidered: A Critical View," *Research in Nursing and Health* 19 (1996): 474; and Secunda, *Women and Their Fathers*, p. 420.

5. Elaine Bell Kaplan, *Not Our Kind of Girl: Unraveling the Myths of Black Teenage Motherhood* (Berkeley: University of California Press, 1997); and Hepburn, "Three-Level Model," pp. 523–534; Patricia Noller and Stephen Bagi, "Parent-Adolescent Communication," *Journal of Adolescence* 8 (1985): 125–44.

6. Secunda, *Women and Their Fathers*, p. 171.

7. See E. Mavis Hetherington and Margaret M. Stanley-Hagan, "The Effects of Divorce on Fathers and Their Children," in *The Role of the Father in Child Development*, 3rd ed., ed. Michael E. Lamb (New York: John Wiley and Sons, 1997), pp. 191–211; Judith S. Wallerstein and Sandra Blakeslee, *Second Chances: Men, Women and Children a Decade after Divorce*, 2nd ed. (Boston: Houghton Mifflin, 1996).

8. Debold, Wilson, and Malavé, *Mother-Daughter Revolution*, p. 232–33.

9. Lamb, *Role of the Father*, pp. 191–211.

10. Derek Davis, "My Daughter's Present," *Philadelphia Forum* 2, no. 19 (June 12, 1997): 1, 5.

11. Debold, Wilson, Malavé, *Mother-Daughter Revolution*, p. 235.

## 10: GETTING IT RIGHT: MATERNAL STRATEGIES

1. Ellen Goodman, "Trusting Mother's New Little Helper," *Philadelphia Inquirer*, February 17, 1997, p. A15.

2. U.S. Department of Health and Human Services, *Fertility, Family Planning, and Women's Health*, p. 30. Moore, *Facts at a Glance*; Brown and Eisenberg, *Best Intentions*, p. 96; Carnegie Council, *Great Transitions*, p. 24.

## AFTERWORD: BEYOND THE FAMILY: INVOLVING THE COMMUNITY

1. *Planned Parenthood Fact Sheet: Sexuality Education in the United States* (New York: Planned Parenthood Federation of America, June 1993), p. 1; Stanley M. Elam, Lowell C. Rose, and Alec M. Gallup, "The 19th Annual Gallup/Phi Delta Kappa Poll of the Public's Attitudes toward the Public Schools," *Phi Delta Kappa*, September 1987, p. 12; Stanley M. Elam, Lowell C. Rose, and Alec M. Gallup, "The 24th Annual Gallup/Phi Delta Kappa Poll of the Public's Attitudes toward the Public Schools," *Phi Delta Kappa*, September 1992, pp. 43–44.

2. Paula Braverman, "The Practitioner's Role," *Clinical Pediatrics* 2 (1994): 100; Mark A. Schuster et al., "Communication between Adolescents and Physicians about Sexual Behavior and Risk Prevention," *Archives of Pediatric Adolescent Medicine* 150 (September 1996): 906–13.

3. Task Force on Pediatric Education, *The Future of Pediatric Education* (Evanston, Ill.: American Academy of Pediatrics, 1978); Esther H. Wender, Polly E. Bijur, and W. Thomas Boyce, "Pediatric Residency Training: Ten Years after the

Task Force Report," *Pediatrics* 90 (1992):876–80; Braverman, "Practitioner's Role," 109.

4. On the Los Angeles study, see Schuster et al., "Communication between Adolescents and Physicians," 911–12; study of adolescents consulting health care providers: Bradley O. Boekeloo et al., "Young Adolescents' Comfort with Discussion about Sexual Problems with Their Physician," *Archives of Pediatric Adolescent Medicine* 150 (November 1996): 1148.

5. Boekeloo et al., "Young Adolescents' Comfort with Discussion," p. 1149.

6. Braverman, "Practitioner's Role," p. 105.

7. Ibid, p. 104.

8. Kirby et al., "School-Based Programs," p. 340.

9. Mark W. Roosa and F. Scott Christopher, "Evaluation of an Abstinence-Only Adolescent Pregnancy Prevention Program: A Replication," *Family Relations* 39 (1990): 363–67; F. Scott Christopher and Mark W. Roosa, "An Evaluation of an Adolescent Pregnancy Prevention Program: Is Just Say No' Enough?" *Family Relations*, January 1990, pp. 68–71; Stephen R. Jorgensen, Vicki Potts, and Brian Camp, "Project Taking Charge: Six-Month Follow-Up of a Pregnancy Prevention Program for Early Adolescents," *Family Relations* 42 (1993): 401–6; Douglas Kirby et al., "The Impact of Postponing Sexual Involvement Curriculum among Youth in California," *Family Planning Perspectives* 29 (1997): 100–108; Kirby et al., "School-Based Programs," p. 352.

10. Kirby et al., "School-Based Programs," pp. 339–59.

11. Ibid.; Roosa and Christopher, "Evaluation of an Abstinence-Only Adolescent Pregnancy Prevention Program," pp. 363–67.

12. Burlingame, *Sex, Lies and Politics*, p. 14.

13. Ibid., pp. 13–14.

14. Ibid., pp. 14, 16.

15. On sex education requirements, see Brown and Eisenberg, *Best Intentions*, p. 132; J. L. Collins et al., "School Health Education," *Journal of School Health* 65, no. 8 (October 1995): 302–11; Sexuality Information and Education Council of the United States, National Guidelines Task Force, *Guidelines for Comprehensive Sexuality Education: Kindergarten through 12th Grade*, 2nd ed. (New York: SIECUS, 1996).

16. "Sexuality Education in the Schools: Issues and Answers," *SIECUS Report* 24, no. 6 (August-September 1996), pp. 1–4; Debra W. Haffner, *Sexual Health for America's Adolescents: The Report of the National Commission on Adolescent Sexual Health, Sexuality Information and Education Council of the U.S.* (New York: SIECUS, 1995).

17. Anita Clark, "State Seeks Money to Teach Abstinence," *Wisconsin State Journal*, June 8, 1997, pp. 1–3.

18. J. Stryker, "Abstinence or Else," *Nation*, June 16, 1997, p. 20.

19. Edith B. Phelps, *No Turning Back: Milestones for Girls in the Twentieth Century* (New York: Girls Inc., 1995), p. 144.

20. B. C. Miller, R. Christensen, and T. D. Olson, "Self-Esteem in Relation to Adolescent Sexual Attitudes and Behavior," *Youth and Society* 2, no. 1 (1987): 93.

# Bibliography

*Adolescent Health*. Vol. 1: *Summary and Policy Options*. Congress of the United States, Office of Technology Assessment, April 1991.

American Association of University Women. *Shortchanging Girls, Shortchanging America: A Call to Action*. Washington, D.C.: American Association of University Women, 1991.

American Medical Association. "America's Adolescents: How Healthy Are They?" *Profiles of Adolescent Health*, series 1, 1990.

Ammerman, Seth D., et al. "Do Adolescents Understand What Physicians Say about Sexuality and Health." *Clinical Pediatrics* (October 1992): 590–95.

Anderson, D. Y., and C. L. Hayes. *Gender, Identity and Self-Esteem*. New York: Springer, 1996.

Anderson, J. E., L. Kann, and D. Holtzman. "HIV/AIDS Knowledge and Sexual Behavior among High School Students." *Family Planning Perspectives* 22, no. 6 (1990): 252–55.

Apter, Terri. *Altered Loves: Mothers and Daughters during Adolescence*. New York: St. Martin's Press, 1990.

Arcana, J. *Our Mothers' Daughters*. Berkeley: Shameless Hussy Press, 1979.

Baker, S. A., S. P. Thalberg, and D. M. Morrison. "Parents' Behavioral Norms as Predictors of Adolescent Sexual Activity and Contraceptive Use." *Adolescence* 23, no. 90 (1988): 265–82.

Barnes, H. L., and D. H. Olson. *Parent-Adolescent Communication*. Family Social Science, University of Minnesota, 1982.

———. "Parent-Adolescent Communication and the Circumplex Model." *Child Development* 56 (1985): 438–47.

Baruch, Grace K., Rosalind C. Barnett, and Caryl Rivers. *Lifeprints: New Patterns of Love and Work for Today's Women*. New York: New American Library, 1984.

Beck, J. Gayle, and Dana K. Davies. "Teen Contraception: A Review of Perspectives and Compliance." *Archives of Sexual Behavior* 16, no. 4 (1987): 337–68.

Belenky, M., B. Clinchy, N. Goldberger, and J. Tarula. *Women's Ways of Knowing*. New York: Basic Books, 1986.

Biglan, A., et al. "Social and Behavioral Factors Associated with High-Risk Sexual Behavior among Adolescents." *Journal of Behavioral Medicine* 13, no. 3 (1990): 245–61.

Bloch, D. "Sex Education Practices of Mothers." *Journal of Sex Education and Therapy* 7 (1972): 7–12.

Boekeloo, Bradley O., Lisa A. Schamus, Tina L. Chang, and Samuel J. Simmons. "Young Adolescents' Comfort with Discussion about Sexual Problems with Their Physician." *Archives of Pediatric Adolescent Medicine* 150 (November 1996): 1146–52.

Boston Women's Health Book Collective. *Ourselves and Our Children.* New York: Random House, 1978.

Boyer, D., and D. Fine. "Sexual Abuse as a Factor in Adolescent Pregnancy and Child Maltreatment." *Family Planning Perspectives* 24 (1992): 4–11.

Braverman, Paula. "The Practitioner's Role." *Clinical Pediatrics* 2 (1994).

Braverman, Paula K., and Victor C. Strasburger. "Sexually Transmitted Diseases." *Clinical Pediatrics* 2 (1994): 26–37.

Brooks-Gunn, Jeanne, and Frank F. Furstenberg. "Adolescent Sexual Behavior." *American Psychologist* 44 (1989): 249–57.

Brooks-Gunn, Jeanne, and D. N. Ruble. "The Development of Menstrual-Related Beliefs and Behaviors during Early Adolescence." *Child Development* 53 (1982): 1567–77.

Brown, Jane D., and Jeanne R. Steele. *Sex and the Mass Media.* Menlo Park, Calif.: Henry J. Kaiser Family Foundation, 1995.

Brown, L. M., and Carol Gilligan, *Meeting at the Crossroads.* New York: Ballantine Books, 1992.

Brown, Sarah S., and Leon Eisenberg, eds. *The Best Intentions: Unintended Pregnancy and the Well-Being of Children and Families.* Washington, D.C.: National Academy Press, 1995.

Brumberg, Joan Jacobs, *The Body Project: An Intimate History of American Girls.* New York: Random House, 1997.

Burlingame, Phyllida. *Sex, Lies and Politics: Abstinence-Only Curricula in California Public Schools. A Joint Report from Public Media Center and the Applied Research Center.* Oakland, Calif.: Applied Research Center, May 1997.

Campbell, D. W. "Family Process and Adolescent Sexuality: The Relationship of Family Functioning, Parent-Adolescent Communication, and Age of the Adolescent to Adolescent Disclosure of Sexuality within the Context of the Mother-Daughter Dyad." *Dissertation Abstracts International* 48, no. 7 (1987): 1–194.

Carnegie Council on Adolescent Development. *Great Transitions: Preparing Adolescents for a New Century.* New York: Carnegie Corporation, 1995.

Center for Disease Control. *HIV/AIDS Surveillance Report: AIDS Cases by Age Group, Exposure Category, and Race/Ethnicity, Reported through April 1989, United States.* Atlanta: Center for Disease Control, 1989.

Center for Disease Control. *Teen Sex Survey Report.* Atlanta: Center for Disease Control, 1992.

Childers, Kim Walsh, and Jane Brown. "Teen Media Awareness Mirrors Upbringing." *Media and Values* 46 (Spring 1989): 9.

Children's Television Workshop. *What Kids Want to Know about Sex and Growing Up.* Los Angeles: Pacific Arts Video Publishing, 1992.

Chilman, Catherine S. *Adolescent Sexuality in a Changing American Society: Social and Psychological Perspectives for the Human Services Professions,* 2nd ed. New York: John Wiley and Sons, 1983.

————. "The Development of Adolescent Sexuality." *Journal of Research and Development in Education* 16, no. 2 (1983): 16–26.

Chodorow, Nancy. *The Reproduction of Mothering: Psychoanalysis and the Sociology of Gender.* Berkeley: University of California Press, 1978.

Christopher, F. Scott, and Mark W. Roosa. "An Evaluation of an Adolescent Pregnancy Prevention Program: Is 'Just Say No' Enough?" *Family Relations* (January 1990): 68–71.

Coleman, Brenda C. "Study Finds Earlier Onset of Puberty for American Girls." *Philadelphia Inquirer,* April 8, 1997.

Coles, Robert, and Geoffrey Stokes. *Sex and the American Teenager.* New York: Harper and Row, 1985.

Collins, P. H. "The Meaning of Motherhood in Black Culture and Black Mother-Daughter Relationships." *Sage: A Scholarly Journal on Black Women* 4, no. 2 (1987): 3–10.

Collins, J. L., et al. "School Health Education." *Journal of School Health* 65, no. 8 (October 1995): 302–11.

Consortium for Research on Black Adolescence. *Black Adolescence: Current Issues and Annotated Bibliography.* Boston: G. K. Hall, 1990.

Coombs, Joan S. "Society Must Take Some Responsibility." *Philadelphia Inquirer,* December 8, 1996.

Crenshaw, Theresa. *The Alchemy of Love and Lust.* New York: Putnam, 1996.

Davis, Derek. "My Daughter's Present." *Philadelphia Forum* 2, no. 19 (June 12, 1997): 1,5.

Debold, Elizabeth, Marie Wilson, and Idelisse Malavé. *Mother-Daughter Revolution: From Betrayal to Power.* New York: Addison-Wesley, 1993.

Demetriou, E., and D. Kaplan. "Adolescent Contraceptive Use and Parental Notification." *American Journal of Disabled Children* 143, no. 10 (1989): 1166–72.

DeSantis, L., and J. T. Thomas. "Parental Attitudes toward Adolescent Sexuality: Transcultural Perspectives." *Nurse Practitioner* 12, no. 8 (1987): 43–48.

DiBlasio, F. "Adolescent Sexuality: Promoting the Search for Hidden Values." *Child Welfare League of America* 68, no. 3 (1989): 331–37.

Dixon, P. *Mothers and Mothering: An Annotated Feminist Bibliography.* New York: Garland, 1991.

Durant, R. H., and J. M. Sanders. "Sexual Behavior and Contraceptive Risk Taking among Sexually Active Adolescent Females." *Journal of Adolescent Health Care* 10, no. 1 (1989): 1–9.

Durant, Robert H., et al. "Tobacco and Alcohol Use Behavior Portrayed in Music Videos: A Content Analysis." *American Journal of Public Health* 87, no. 7 (July 1997): 1131–35.

Elam, Stanley M., Lowell C. Rose, and Alec M. Gallup. "The 19th Annual Gallup/Phi Delta Kappa Poll of the Public's Attitudes toward the Public Schools." *Phi Delta Kappa* (September 1987): p. 12.

———. "The 24th Annual Gallup/Phi Delta Kappa Poll of the Public's Attitudes toward the Public Schools." *Phi Delta Kappa* (September 1992): p. 41–44.

Ellwood, D. *Poor Support: Poverty in the American Family*. New York: Basic Books, 1988.

Eng, Thomas R., and William T. Butler. *The Hidden Epidemic: Confronting Sexually Transmitted Diseases*. Washington, D.C.: National Academy Press, 1996.

Ensminger, M. "Sexual Activity and Problem Behaviors among Black, Urban Adolescents." *Child Development* 61 (1990): 2032–46.

Erikson, Erik. *Childhood and Society*, 2nd ed. New York: W. W. Norton, 1963.

———. *Identity, Youth and Crisis*. New York: W. W. Norton, 1968.

Fashee, Vangie, and Karl Bauman. "Gender Stereotyping and Adolescent Behavior." *Journal of Applied Psychology* 22, no. 20 (1992): 1561–79.

Feldman, S., and G. Elliott. *At the Threshold: The Developing Adolescent*. Cambridge, Mass.: Harvard University Press, 1990.

Fine, Michelle. "Sexuality, Schooling and Adolescent Females: The Missing Discourse of Desire." *Harvard Educational Review* 58, no. 1 (1988): 29–48.

Fine, Michelle, and Nancie Zane. "Bein' Wrapped Too Tight: When Low-Income Women Drop Out of School." In L. Weis, R. Farrar, and H. Petrie, eds., *Dropouts in Schools: Issues, Dilemmas and Solutions*. Albany: State University of New York Press, 1989.

Fisher, T. "An Exploratory Study of Parent-Child Communication about Sex and the Sexual Attitudes of Early, Middle, and Late Adolescents." *Journal of Genetic Psychology* 147 (1986): 543–57.

———. "Parent-Child Communication about Sex and Young Adolescents' Sexual Knowledge and Attitudes." *Adolescence* 21, no. 83 (1986): 517–21.

Flinn, Susan K., and Susan A. Messina. "The Politics of Desire: The Touchy Subject of Success in Sex Education." *Bryn Mawr Alumnae Bulletin* (1996): 12–15.

Fox, G. "The Mother-Adolescent Daughter Relationship as a Sexual Socialization Structure: A Research Review." *Family Relations* 29 (January 1980): 21–28.

———. "The Family's Role in Adolescent Sexual Behavior." In T. Ooms, ed., *Teenage Pregnancy in a Family Context*. Philadelphia: Temple University Press, 1981.

Fox, Greer Litton, and Judith K. Inazu. "Patterns and Outcomes of Mother-Daughter Communication about Sexuality." *Journal of Social Issues* 36, no. 1 (1980): 7–29.

Fox, Greer Litton, and C. Medlin. "Accuracy in Mothers' Perceptions of Daughters' Level of Sexual Involvement: Black and White Single Mothers and Their Teenage Daughters." *Family Perspectives* 20 (1986): 267–86.

Fraser, A. M., J. E. Brockert, and R. H. Ward. "Association of Young Maternal Age with Adverse Reproductive Outcomes." *New England Journal of Medicine* 332, no. 17 (1995): 1113–17.

Freud, Sigmund. "Three Essays on the Theory of Sexuality." In James Strachey, ed. and trans., *The Complete Psychological Works of Sigmund Freud*. Vol. 7. London: Hogarth Press, 1905.

Friday, Nancy. *The Power of Beauty*. New York: Harper Collins, 1996.

Furstenberg, F. *Unplanned Parenthood: The Social Consequences of Teenage Childbearing*. New York: Free Press, 1976.

———. "Children's Names and Paternal Claims: Bonds between Unmarried Fathers and Their Children." *Journal of Family Issues* 1 (1979): 21–57.

Furstenberg, Frank, Jr., R. Lincoln, and J. Menken, eds. *Teenage Sexuality, Pregnancy and Childbearing.* Philadelphia: University of Pennsylvania Press, 1981.

Furstenberg, Frank, Jeanne Brooks-Gunn, and L. Chase-Lansdale. "Teenage Pregnancy and Childbearing." *American Psychologist* 44(2) (1989): 313–20.

Furstenberg, Frank, Jeanne Brooks-Gunn, and S. Morgan. "Adolescent Mothers and Their Children in Later Life." *Family Planning Perspectives* 19, no. 4 (1987).

Gilligan, Carol. "In a Different Voice: Women's Conceptions of the Self and of Morality." *Harvard Educational Review* 47 (1977): 481–517.

———. *In a Different Voice: Psychological Theory and Women's Development.* Cambridge, Mass.: Harvard University Press, 1982.

———. "Remapping the Moral Domain: New Images of Self in Relationship." In Carol Gilligan, J. Ward, and J. Taylor, eds., *Mapping the Moral Domain.* Cambridge, Mass.: Harvard University Press, 1988.

Gilligan, Carol, Naomi P. Lyons, and Trudy J. Hanmer. *Making Connections: The Relational Worlds of Adolescent Girls at Emma Willard School.* Cambridge, Mass.: Harvard University Press, 1990.

Haffner, Debra W. *Sexual Health for America's Adolescents: The Report of the National Commission on Adolescent Sexual Health, Sexuality Information and Education Council of the United States.* New York: SIECUS, 1995.

Hakim, P., J. Larson, and C. Hobard. "Maternal Regulation and Adolescent Autonomy: Mother-Daughter Resolution of Story Conflicts." *Journal of Youth and Adolescence* 16, no. 2 (1987): 153–66.

Hammer, Signe. *Daughters and Mothers: Mothers and Daughters.* New York: New York Times Books, 1975.

Hartman, Lauren. *Solutions: The Woman's Crisis Handbook.* Boston: Houghton Mifflin, 1997.

Hatcher, Robert A., et al. *Contraceptive Technology: 1990–1992.* 15th ed. New York: Irvington, 1990.

Hepburn, Eileen. "A Three-Level Model of Parent-Daughter Communication about Sexual Topics." *Adolescence* 18, no. 71 (1983): 523–34.

Herman-Giddens, Marcia E., et al. "Secondary Sexual Characteristics and Menses in Young Girls Seen in Office Practice: A Study from the Pediatric Research in Office Settings Network." *Pediatrics* 99, no. 4 (April 1997): 505–12.

Heron, Ann, ed. *Two Teenagers in Twenty: Writings by Gay and Lesbian Youth.* Los Angeles: Alyson Publications, 1983; reprint, Ann Heron, 1994.

Hetherington, E. Mavis, and Margaret M. Stanley-Hagan. "The Effects of Divorce on Fathers and Their Children." In *The Role of the Father in Child Development,* 3rd ed., ed. Michael E. Lamb. New York: John Wiley and Sons, 1997.

Heyn, Delma. *The Erotic Silence of the American Wife.* New York: Random House, 1992.

Hite, Shere. *The Hite Report: A Nationwide Study of Female Sexuality.* New York: Dell, 1976.

Hockenberry-Eaton, Marilyn, et al. "Mother and Adolescent Knowledge of Sexual Development: The Effect of Gender, Age and Sexual Experience." *Adolescence* 31, no. 121 (1996): 35–47.

Horn, M., and Rudolph, L. "An Investigation of Verbal Interaction, Knowledge of Sexual Behavior and Self-Concept in Adolescent Mothers." *Adolescence* 22, no. 87 (1987): 591–98.

Inazu, Judith K., and Greer Litton Fox. "Maternal Influence on the Sexual Behaviors of Teenage Daughters." *Journal of Family Issues* 1, no. 1 (1980): 81–102.

Inhelder, B., and Jean Piaget. *The Growth of Logical Thinking from Childhood to Adolescence*. New York: Basic Books, 1958.

Jaccard, James, Patricia J. Dittus, and Vivian V. Gordon. "Maternal Correlates of Adolescent Sexual and Contraceptive Behavior." *Family Planning Perspectives* 28, no. 4 (July/August 1996): 159–85.

Jessor, R. "Problem-Behavior Theory, Psychosocial Development, and Adolescent Problem Drinking." *British Journal of Addiction* 82 (1987): 331–42.

Jessor, R., F. Costa, L. Jessor, and J. Donovan. "Time of First Intercourse: A Prospective Study." *Journal of Personality and Social Psychology* 44, no. 3 (1983): 608–26.

Johnson, Lloyd D., Patrick M. O'Malley, and Jerald G. Bachman. *National Survey Results on Drug Use from the Monitoring the Future Study, 1975–1994.* Rockville, Md.: U.S. Department of Health and Human Services, Public Health Service, National Institutes of Health, National Institute on Drug Use, 1995.

Jorgensen, S. "Beyond Adolescent Pregnancy: Research Frontiers for Early Adolescent Sexuality." *Journal of Early Adolescence* 3, nos. 1–2 (1983): 141–55.

Jorgensen, Stephen R., Vicki Potts, and Brian Camp. "Project Taking Charge: Six-Month Follow-up of a Pregnancy Prevention Program for Early Adolescents." *Family Relations* 42 (1993): 401–6.

Joseph, G. "Mothers and Daughters: Traditional and New Perspectives." *Sage: A Scholarly Journal on Black Women* 1, no. 2 (1984): 17–21.

Juhasz, A., and M. Sonnenshein-Schneider. "Adolescent Sexual Decision Making: Components and Skills." *Adolescence* 15, no. 60 (1980): 743–50.

———. "Adolescent Sexuality: Values, Morality and Decision Making." *Adolescence* 22, no. 87 (1987): 579–90.

Kaiser Family Foundation. *Sex, Kids and the Family Hour: A Three-Part Study of Sexual Content on Television*. Menlo Park, Calif.: Henry J. Kaiser Family Foundation, 1996.

*Kaiser Family Foundation Survey on Teens and Sex: What They Say Teens Need to Know and Who They Listen To*. Princeton, N.J.: Survey Research Associates, June 24, 1996.

Kaplan, Elaine Bell. *Not Our Kind of Girl: Unraveling the Myths of Black Teenage Motherhood*. Berkeley: University of California Press, 1997.

Kantner, J., M. and M. Zelnik. "Sexual Experience of Young Unmarried Women in the United States." *Family Planning Perspectives* 5, no. 1 (1972): 11–25.

Kastner, Laura S., and Jennifer F. Wyatt. *The Seven-Year Stretch: How Families Work Together to Grow through Adolescence*. Boston: Houghton Mifflin, 1997.

Kenny, A. M., S. Guardado, and L. Brown. "Sex Education and AIDS Education in the Schools: What States and Large School Districts Are Doing." *Family Planning Perspectives* 21, no. 2 (1989): 56–64.

Kinnard, K. L., and M. Gerrard. "Premarital Sexual Behavior and Attitudes toward Marriage and Divorce among Young Women as a Function of Their Mothers' Marital Status." *Journal of Marriage and the Family* 48 (1986): 757–85.

Kirby, Douglas, et al. "School-Based Programs to Reduce Sexual Risk Behaviors: A Review of Effectiveness." *Public Health Reports* 109, no. 3 (May-June 1994): 339–59.

————. "The Impact of Postponing Sexual Involvement Curriculum among Youth in California." *Family Planning Perspectives* 29 (1997): 100–108.

Koff, Elissa, and Jill Rierdan. "Preparing Girls for Menstruation: Recommendations from Adolescent Girls. *Adolescence* 30, no. 120 (Winter 1995): 795–811.

————. "Early Adolescent Girls' Understanding of Menstruation." *Women and Health* 22, no. 4 (1995): 1–19.

Koppelman, S. *Between Mothers and Daughters: Stories across a Generation.* New York: Feminist Press, 1985.

Koppleman, J. "Reducing Teen Pregnancy and Childbearing in America: What is the Federal Role?" *National Health Policy Forum*, Issue Brief 654 (1995).

Ladner, J. A., and R. M. Gourdine. "Intergenerational Teenage Motherhood: Some Preliminary Findings." *Sage: A Scholarly Journal on Black Women* 1, no 2 (1984): 22–24.

Lamb, M., ed. *The Role of the Father in Child Development*, 3rd ed. New York: John Wiley and Sons, 1997.

Landry, David J. and Jacqueline D. Forrest. "How Old Are U.S. Fathers?" *Family Planning Perspectives* 27, no. 4 (1995): 159–61, 165.

Larson, R. W. "Finding Time for Fatherhood: The Emotional Ecology of Adolescent-Father Interactions." In S. Shulman and W. A. Collins, eds., *Father-Adolescent Relationships: New Directions for Childhood.* San Francisco: Jossey-Bass, 1993.

LeVine, Robert. "Human Parental Care: Universal Goals, Cultural Strategies, Individual Behavior." In Robert A. LeVine, P. M. Miller, and M. M. West, eds. *New Directions for Child Development: Parental Behavior in Diverse Societies.* San Francisco: Jossey-Bass, 1988.

Lichter, S. Robert, Linda S. Lichter, and Stanley Rothman. *Prime Time: How TV Portrays American Culture.* Washington, D.C.: Regency Publishing, 1994.

Lightfoot, Sara Lawrence. *Balm in Gilead: Journey of a Healer.* Reading, Mass.: Addison-Wesley, 1988.

Lindegren, Mary Lou, et al. "Epidemiology of Human Immunodeficiency Virus Infection in Adolescents, United States." *Pediatric Infectious Diseases Journal* 13 (1994): 525–35.

Lipton, E. "Representing Sexuality in Women Artists' Biographies: The Cases of Suzanne Valadon and Victorine." *Journal of Sex Research* 27, no. 1 (1990): 81-94.

Luker, Kristin. *Dubious Conceptions: The Politics of Teenage Pregnancy.* Cambridge, Mass.: Harvard University Press, 1996.

Males, Mike, and Kenneth Chew. "The Age of Fathers in California Adolescent Births, 1993." *American Journal of Public Health* 84, no. 4 (April 1996): 565–68.

Miller, Brent C. "Adolescents' Relationships with Their Friends." Doctoral dissertation, Harvard Graduate School of Education, 1991.

Miller, Brent C., and Greer Litton Fox. "Theories of Adolescent Heterosexual Behavior." *Journal of Adolescent Research* 2, no. 3 (1987): 269–82.

Miller, Brent C., R. Christensen, and T. D. Olson, "Self-Esteem in Relation to Adolescent Sexual Attitudes and Behavior." *Youth and Society* 2, no. 1 (1987): 93.

Miller, Jean Baker. *Toward a New Psychology of Women.* Boston: Beacon Press, 1976; rev. ed., 1986.

Minow, Newton N., and C. L. Lamay. *Abandoned in the Wasteland: Children, Television and the First Amendment.* New York: Hill and Wang, 1995.

Montemayor, R., M. Eberly, and D. J. Flannery. "Effects of Pubertal Status and Conversation Topic on Parent and Adolescent Affective Expression." *Journal of Early Adolescence* 13 (1993): 431–47.

Moore, Kristin A. *Facts at a Glance.* Washington, D.C.: Child Trends, January 1996.

Moore, Kristin A., J. Peterson, and Frank F. Furstenberg. "Parental Attitudes and the Occurrence of Early Sexual Activity." *Journal of Marriage and the Family* 48, no. 4 (1986): 777–82.

Moore, Kristin A., M. Simms, and C. Betsy. *Choice and Circumstances: Racial Differences in Adolescent Sexuality and Fertility.* New Brunswick, N.J.: Transition Books, 1986.

Mueller, K., and W. Powers. "Parent-Child Sexual Discussion: Perceived Communicator Style and Subsequent Behavior." *Adolescence* 25, no. 98 (1990): 469–82.

Newcomer, Susan F., and J. Richard Udry. "Mothers' Influence on the Sexual Behavior of Their Teenage Children." *Journal of Marriage and the Family* 46 (1984): 477–85.

———. "Parent-Child Communication and Adolescent Sexual Behavior." *Family Planning Perspectives* 417 (1985): 169–74.

Noller, Patricia, and Stephen Bagi. "Parent-Adolescent Communication." *Journal of Adolescence* 8, no. 2 (1985): 125–44.

Olsen, Tillie. *Mother to Daughter, Daughter to Mother, Mothers on Mothering.* New York: Feminist Press, 1984.

Orenstein, Peggy. *School Girls: Young Women, Self-Esteem and the Confidence Gap.* New York: Doubleday, 1994.

Pete, J., and L. DeSantis. "Sexual Decision Making in Young Black Adolescent Females." *Adolescence* 25, no. 97 (1990): 145–54.

Phelps, Edith B. *No Turning Back: Milestones for Girls in the Twentieth Century.* New York: Girls Inc., 1995.

Pipher, Mary. *Reviving Ophelia: Saving the Selves of Adolescent Girls.* New York: Ballantine Books, 1994.

*Planned Parenthood Fact Sheet: Sexuality Education in the United States.* New York: Planned Parenthood Federation of America, June 1993.

Pratt, J., and K. Pryor. *About America's Teenagers.* New York: Hyperion, 1995.

Rafkin, Louise, ed. *Different Daughters: A Book by Mothers of Lesbians,* 2nd ed. Pittsburgh: Cleis Press, 1987.

Resnick, Michael D., et al. "Protecting Adolescents from Harm: Findings from the National Longitudinal Study on Adolescent Health. *Journal of the American Medical Association* 278, no. 10 (Sept 10, 1997): 823–32.

Rich, Adrienne. *Of Woman Born: Motherhood as Experience and Institution*. New York: W. W. Norton, 1976.

Rich, Sharon. "Change within Connection: A Study of Adolescent Daughters' Views of Their Relationship with Their Mothers." Doctoral dissertation, Harvard Graduate School of Education, 1986.

Richmond, J. "Human Development." In B. Jones, ed., *The Health of Americans: The American Assembly, Columbia University*. Englewood Cliffs, N.J.: Prentice-Hall, 1970.

Roberts, E. J. *Children's Sexual Learning: An Examination of the Influence of Parents, Television, and Community Service Providers*. Doctoral dissertation, Harvard Graduate School of Education, 1982.

Roosa, Mark W., and F. Scott Christopher. "Evaluation of an Abstinence-Only Adolescent Pregnancy Prevention Program: A Replication." *Family Relations* 39 (1990): 363–67.

Rosen, R. "Adolescent Pregnancy Decision Making: Are Parents Important?" *Adolescence* 15, no. 57 (1980): 43–54.

Rothenberg, P. "Communication about Sex and Birth Control between Mothers and Their Adolescent Children." *Population and Environment* 3 (Spring 1980): 35–50.

Rotheram-Borus, Mary J., and Fernandez, M. Isabela. "Sexual Orientation and Developmental Challenges Experienced by Gay and Lesbian Youths." *Suicide and Life-Threatening Behavior* 25, suppl. (1995): 26–39.

Ruddick, S. *Maternal Thinking*. Boston: Beacon Press, 1989.

Ryan, Caitlin, and Dona Futterman. "Overview: HIV Infection in Adolescents Including Lesbians and Gay Males." In *Lesbian and Gay Youth: Care and Counseling*. Philadelphia: Hanley and Belfus, 1997.

Sander, J. *Before Their Time*. New York: Harcourt Brace Jovanovich, 1991.

Savin-Williams, R., and S. Small. "The Timing of Puberty and Its Relationship to Adolescent and Parent Perceptions of Family Interactions." *Developmental Psychology* 22, no. 3 (1986): 342–47.

Schorr, Lisbeth. *Within Our Reach: Breaking the Cycle of Disadvantage*. New York: Doubleday, 1988.

Schuster, Mark A., et al. "Communication between Adolescents and Physicians about Sexual Behavior and Risk Prevention." *Archives of Pediatric Adolescent Medicine* 150 (September 1996): 906–13.

Schuster, Mark A., Robert M. Bell, and David E. Kanouse. "The Sexual Practices of Adolescent Virgins: Genital Sexual Activities of High School Graduate Students Who Have Never Had Sexual Intercourse." *American Journal of Public Health* 86, no. 11 (November 1996): 1570–76.

Secunda, Victoria. *Women and Their Fathers: The Sexual and Romantic Impact of the First Man in Your Life*. New York: Delacorte Press, 1992.

Sells, C. Wayne, and Robert W. Blum. "Morbidity and Mortality among U.S. Adolescents: An Overview of Data and Trends." *American Journal of Public Health* 86, no. 4 (April 1996): 513–19.

*Sex and America's Teenagers*. New York: Alan Guttmacher Institute, 1994.

Sexuality Information and Education Council of the United States, National Guidelines Task Force. *Guidelines for Comprehensive Sexuality Education: Kindergarten through 12th Grade*, 2nd ed. New York: SIECUS, 1996.

Shah, F., and M. Zelnik. "Parent and Peer Influence on Sexual Behavior, Contraceptive Use and Pregnancy Experience of Young Women." *Journal of Marriage and the Family* 43 (1981): 339–48.

Sidel, R. *On Her Own.* New York: Viking Penguin, 1990.

Silverberg, S., and L. Steinberg. "Psychological Well-Being of Parents with Early Adolescent Children." *Developmental Psychology* 26, no. 4 (1990): 658–66.

Simmons, Roberta G., and Dale A. Blyth. *Moving into Adolescence: The Impact of Pubertal Change and School Context.* Hawthorne, N.Y.: Aldine De Gruyter, 1987.

Smith, E., and J. Udry. "Coital and Non-Coital Sexual Behaviors of White and Black Adolescents." *American Journal of Public Health* 75, no. 10 (1985): 1200–1203.

Smith, M. O., and D. Smith-Blackmer. "The Mother-Daughter Relationship: A Dialogue Continued." *Clinical Social Work Journal* 9, no. 1 (1981): 57–68.

Smollar, J., and J. Youniss. "Parent-Adolescent Relations in Adolescents Whose Parents Are Divorced." *Journal of Early Adolescence* 5 (1985): 129–44.

Spitz, Alison M., et al. "Pregnancy, Abortion and Birth Rates among U.S. Adolescents — 1980, 1985 and 1990." *Journal of the American Medical Association* 275, no. 13 (April 3, 1996): 989–94.

*State of America's Children: Yearbook 1997.* Washington, D.C.: Children's Defense Fund, 1997.

Steinberg, L. "The Impact of Puberty on Family Relations: Effects of Pubertal Status and Pubertal Timing." *Developmental Psychology* 23 (1987): 451–60.

———. "Autonomy, Conflict and Harmony in the Family Relationship." In S. Feldman and G. Elliott, eds., *At the Threshold: The Developing Adolescent.* Cambridge, Mass.: Harvard University Press, 1990.

Steinhauer, Jennifer. "Study Cites Adult Males for the Most Teen-Age Births." *New York Times,* August 2, 1995.

Stevens-Simon, Catherine, and Susan Reichert. "Sexual Abuse, Adolescent Pregnancy and Child Abuse: A Developmental Approach to an Intergenerational Cycle." *Archives of Pediatrics and Adolescent Medicine* 148, no. 1 (January 1994): 23–27.

Stiver, I. P. "Beyond the Oedipus Complex: Mothers and Daughters." Working paper no. 26. Stone Center for Developmental Services and Studies, Wellesley College, 1986.

Strasburger, Victor C. *Adolescents and the Media: Medical and Psychological Impact.* Thousand Oaks, Calif.: Sage Publications, 1995.

———. "Children, Adolescents and Television." *Pediatrics in Review* 13, no. 4 (April 1992): 144–51.

Stryker, J. "Abstinence or Else." *Nation,* June 16, 1997, p. 20.

Stubbs, Margaret L., Jill Rierdan, and Elissa Koff. "Becoming a Woman: Considerations in Educating Adolescents about Menstruation." Working paper no. 169. Center for Research on Women, Wellesley College, 1988.

Swan, R. "Communicating about Sexuality in Catholic Homes." *Journal of Social Work and Human Sexuality* 1, no. 3 (1983): 39–52.

Task Force on Pediatric Education. *The Future of Pediatric Education.* Evanston, Ill.: American Academy of Pediatrics, 1978.

Thompson, Sharon. "Search for Tomorrow: On Feminism and the Reconstruction of Teen Romance." In Carol Vance, ed., *Pleasure and Danger: Exploring Female Sexuality*. Boston: Routledge and Kegan Paul, 1984.

————. "Putting a Big Thing into a Little Hole: Teenage Girls' Accounts of Sexual Initiation." *Journal of Sex Research* 27, no. 1 (1990): 81–94.

————. *Going All the Way: Teenage Girls' Tales of Sex, Romance and Pregnancy*. New York: Hill and Wang, 1995.

Tiedje, Linda Beth, and Cynthia Darling-Fisher. "Fatherhood Reconsidered: A Critical View." *Research in Nursing and Health* 19 (1996): 471–84.

Tolman, Deborah L. "Discourses of Adolescent Girls' Sexual Desire in Developmental Psychology and Feminist Scholarship." Qualifying paper, Harvard Graduate School of Education, 1990.

Tolman, Deborah L., and Tracy E. Higgins. "How Being a Good Girl Can Be Bad for Girls." In Nan Bauer Maglin and Donna Perry, eds., *Bad Girls, Good Girls: Women, Sex and Power in the Nineties*. New Brunswick, N.J.: Rutgers University Press, 1996.

U.S. Department of Health and Human Services, Center for Disease Control and Prevention, National Center for Health Statistics. *Vital and Health Statistics. Fertility, Family Planning and Women's Health: New Data from the 1995 National Survey on Family Growth*. Series 23, no. 19 (May 1997), DHHS publication no. (PHS) 97–1995.

U.S. General Accounting Office. *Welfare Dependency: Coordinated Efforts Can Better Serve Young At-Risk Teen Girls*. GAO/HEH/RCED–95–108. Washington, D.C.: U.S. General Accounting Office, 1995.

U.S. House of Representatives. *U.S. Children and Their Families: Current Conditions and Recent Trends*. Washington, D.C.: U.S. Government Printing Office, 1989.

Udry, J., L. Talbert, and N. Morris. "Biosocial Foundations for Adolescent Female Sexuality." *Demography* 23, no. 2 (1986): 217–27.

Vance, Carol S., and Carol A. Pollis. "Introduction: A Special Issue on Feminist Perspectives in Sexuality." *Journal of Sex Research* 27, no. 1 (1990): 1–5.

Vanderpool, N. A. "Communication between Mothers and Adolescent Daughters on Issues of Sexuality: A Literature Review." Qualifying paper, Harvard Graduate School of Education, 1991.

————. "Young Children and Families: Creating a Social Policy Agenda: A Review of Selected Reports." Background paper for Task Force on Meeting the Needs of Young Children. Carnegie Corporation of New York, 1993.

Vanderpool, N. A., and J. Richmond. "Child Health in the United States: Prospects for the 1990s." *Annual Review of Public Health* 11 (1990): 185–205.

Wallerstein, Judith S., and Sandra Blakeslee. *Second Chances: Men, Women and Children a Decade after Divorce*. Boston: Houghton Mifflin, 1996.

Walters, J., and L. Walters. "The Role of the Family in Sex Education." *Journal of Research and Development in Education* 16 (1983): 8–15.

Ward, L. Monique. "Talking about Sex: Common Themes about Sexuality in the Prime Time Television Programs Children and Adolescents View Most." *Journal of Youth and Adolescence* 24, no. 5 (1995): 595–615.

Webster, Paula. "The Forbidden Eroticism and Taboo." In Carole S. Vance, ed., *Pleasure and Danger: Exploring Female Sexuality*. Boston: Routledge and Kegan Paul, 1984.

Weddle, K., P. McHenry, and G. Leigh. "Adolescent Sexual Behavior: Trends and Issues in Research." *Journal of Adolescent Research* 3, nos. 3–4. (1988): 245–57.

Weinstein, M., and A. Thornton. "Mother-Child Relations and Adolescent Sexual Attitudes and Behavior." *Demography* 26, no. 4 (1989): 563–77.

Wender, Esther H., Polly E. Bijur, and W. Thomas Boyce. "Pediatric Residency Training: Ten Years after the Task Force Report." *Pediatrics* 90 (1992): 876–80.

Whisnant, Lynn, and Leonard Zegans. "A Study of Attitudes toward Menarche in White Middle-Class American Adolescent Girls." *Journal of Psychiatry* 132, no. 8 (1975): 809–14.

Whitfield, M. "Development of Sexuality in Female Children and Adolescents." *Canadian Journal of Psychiatry* 34 (1989): 879–83.

Whiting, B. B. *Children of Different Worlds*. Cambridge, Mass.: Harvard University Press, 1988.

Willie, C. *Black and White Families*. Dix Hill, N.Y.: General Hall, 1988.

Wolf, Naomi. *Promiscuities: The Secret Struggle for Womanhood*. New York: Random House, 1997.

Yalom, M., S. Estler, and W. Brewster. "Changes in Female Sexuality: A Study of Mother-Daughter Communication and Generational Differences." *Psychology of Women Quarterly*, 7, no. 2 (1982): 141–54.

Youniss, J., and R. D. Ketterlinus. "Communication and Connectedness in Mother and Father-Adolescent Relationships." *Journal of Youth and Adolescence* 16 (1987): 265–80.

Zelnik, M., and Shah, F. "First Intercourse among Young Americans." *Family Planning Perspectives* 15, no. 2 (1983): 64–70.

Zelnik, M., J. Kantner, and K. Ford. *Sex and Pregnancy in Adolescence*. Beverly Hills, Calif.: Sage, 1981.

# Index